Edition

BEST △ TENT
Camping

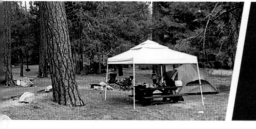

Southern
CALIFORNIA

YOUR CAR-CAMPING GUIDE TO SCENIC BEAUTY, THE SOUNDS
OF NATURE, AND AN ESCAPE FROM CIVILIZATION

Best Tent Camping: Southern California
Fifth edition, second printing 2018
Copyright © 2008 and 2018 Charles Patterson
Copyright © 1996, 2001, 2004 Bill Mai
All rights reserved
Published by Menasha Ridge Press
Distributed by Publishers Group West
Printed in China

Library of Congress Cataloging-in-Publication Data

Names: Patterson, Charles Falk, author.
Title: Best tent camping Southern California : your car-camping guide to
  scenic beauty, the sounds of nature, and an escape from civilization /
  Charles Patterson.
Description: 5th edition. | Birmingham, AL : Menasha Ridge Press, An imprint
  of AdventureKEEN, [2017] | Includes index. | Revised edition of: The best
  in tent camping, Southern California / Charles Falk Patterson and Bill
  Mai. 4th edition. c2010.
Identifiers: LCCN 2017044116| ISBN 9781634040464 (pbk.) | ISBN 9781634040471
  (ebook)
Subjects: LCSH: Camping—California, Southern—Guidebooks. | Camp sites,
  facilities, etc.—California, Southern—Guidebooks. | California,
  Southern—Guidebooks.
Classification: LCC GV191.42.C2 P38 2017 | DDC 917.94/068—dc23
LC record available at https://lccn.loc.gov/2017044116

Cover and interior design: Jonathan Norberg
Cover photo: © James Kaiser; inset photo: © U.S. Department of Agriculture
Photos: Shutterstock (pages 137, 138, 140, 146, and 147). All others are noted on page.
Maps: Steve Jones and Charles Patterson
Indexing: Rich Carlson

MENASHA RIDGE PRESS

An imprint of AdventureKEEN
2204 First Ave. S., Ste. 102
Birmingham, AL 35233

Visit menasharidge.com for a complete listing of our books and for ordering information. Contact us at our website, at facebook.com/menasharidge, or at twitter.com/menasharidge with questions or comments. To find out more about who we are and what we're doing, visit blog.menasharidge.com.

Front cover: Main photo: Joshua Tree National Park: White Tank Campground
Inset photo: Hanna Flat Family Campground

5TH Edition

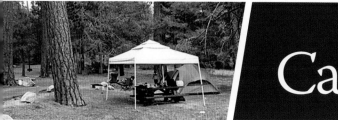

BEST TENT Camping

Southern
CALIFORNIA

YOUR CAR-CAMPING GUIDE TO SCENIC BEAUTY, THE SOUNDS
OF NATURE, AND AN ESCAPE FROM CIVILIZATION

Charles Patterson

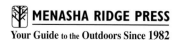

MENASHA RIDGE PRESS
Your Guide to the Outdoors Since 1982

Southern California Campground Locator Map

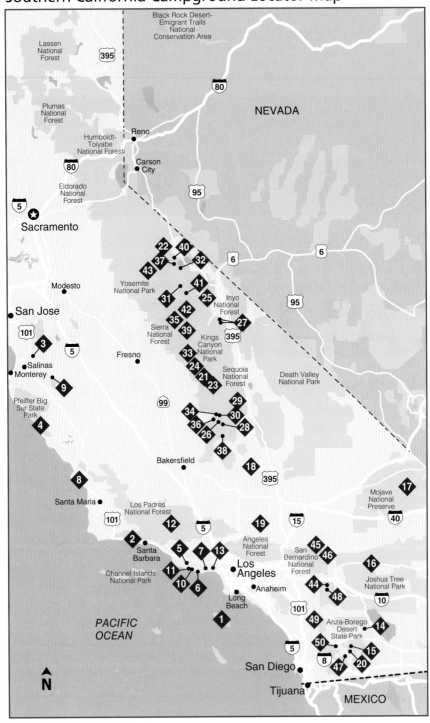

CONTENTS

Map Legend

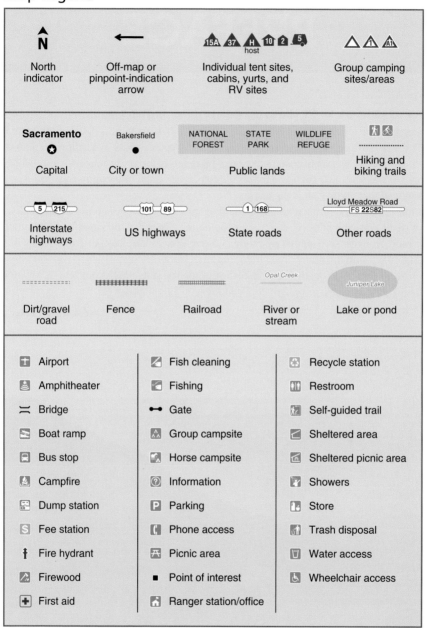

North indicator

Off-map or pinpoint-indication arrow

Individual tent sites, cabins, yurts, and RV sites
15A 37 H host 10 2 5

Group camping sites/areas

Sacramento
Capital

Bakersfield
City or town

NATIONAL FOREST   STATE PARK   WILDLIFE REFUGE
Public lands

Hiking and biking trails

Interstate highways
5 215

US highways
101 89

State roads
1 168

Other roads
Lloyd Meadow Road
FS 22S82

Dirt/gravel road

Fence

Railroad

River or stream
Opal Creek

Lake or pond
Juniper Lake

- ✝ Airport
- 🍺 Amphitheater
- ⟊ Bridge
- 🛥 Boat ramp
- 🚌 Bus stop
- 🔥 Campfire
- Dump station
- Ⓢ Fee station
- ✦ Fire hydrant
- Firewood
- ✚ First aid

- Fish cleaning
- Fishing
- •— Gate
- Group campsite
- Horse campsite
- ⓘ Information
- Ⓟ Parking
- Phone access
- 🏕 Picnic area
- ▪ Point of interest
- Ranger station/office

- ♻ Recycle station
- Restroom
- Self-guided trail
- Sheltered area
- Sheltered picnic area
- Showers
- Store
- Trash disposal
- Water access
- ♿ Wheelchair access

PREFACE

Outdoor adventurers in 49 states will surely protest this, but I must say it—California is the best state for tent camping. Although every state has its natural delights, no state has the variety of outdoor experiences and environments you can find by visiting the sites outlined in this book. What other state has great places to camp on beaches, in alpine forests, dreamy coastal foothills, surreal Martian desert landscapes, and balmy offshore islands? Not one, and that's why Cali is the champ.

In this book, you'll find a wide assortment of sites in a variety of areas. Visit even a fraction of them and your life will change for the better. We're far too separated from nature in our modern lives, surrounded by modern conveniences that keep us from being "in the moment." We spend too many hours indoors and in front of screens these days. Get outside! There's no better way to destress and refresh your mental state. Pitch your tent. Climb. Ride. Fish. Hunt. Hike. Or just sit on a rock. Trust me, you'll be happier.

—Charles Patterson

Savor the beauty of Anza-Borrego Desert State Park near Blair Valley (see page 53).

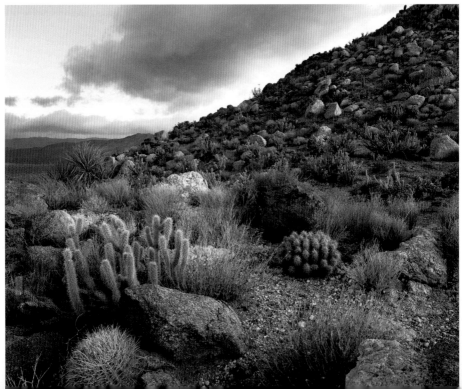

photographed by Bob Carroll

BEST CAMPGROUNDS

BEST FOR PADDLING

BEST FOR PRIVACY

BEST FOR SECURITY

BEST FOR SWIMMING

BEST FOR WHEELCHAIRS

INTRODUCTION

HOW TO USE THIS GUIDEBOOK

Menasha Ridge Press welcomes you to *Best Tent Camping: Southern California*. Whether you are new to this activity or have been sleeping in your portable outdoor shelter during decades of outdoor adventures, please review the following information. It explains how we have worked with the author to organize this book and how you can make the best use of it.

THE RATINGS SYSTEM

As with all books in the Best Tent Camping series, the author personally experienced dozens of campgrounds and campsites to select the top 50 locations in Southern California. Within that universe of 50 sites, the author then ranked each one in the six categories described below.

Each campground is superlative in its own way. For example, a site may be rated only one star in category but perhaps five stars in another category. Our rating system allows you to choose your destination based on the attributes that are most important to you. Although these ratings are subjective, they're still excellent guidelines for finding the perfect camping experience for you and your companions.

★★★★★   The site is **ideal** in that category.

★★★★   The site is **exemplary** in that category.

★★★   The site is **very good** in that category.

★★   The site is **above average** in that category.

★   The site is **acceptable** in that category.

BEAUTY

While all the campgrounds in this book are beautiful, some are absolutely sensational. They rate five stars, with mountains, streams, waterfalls, and sunsets all conspiring for a drop-dead campground personality. One- to four-star campgrounds possess a less-spectacular beauty that will grow on you.

PRIVACY

Some campgrounds are very well built. The sites are arranged to take maximum advantage of the contour of the land, and the vegetation gives each one the most privacy possible. Good architecture cuts down on the cringe factor when other campers pull in next door. It makes you feel at home from the moment you step out of your car. What a difference!

SPACIOUSNESS

I want flat land to pitch a tent on. I want the flat area to be far enough away from the picnic table so my camping mate can make coffee without waking me and far enough away from the fire pit so the embers don't burn holes in the tent. And I want a view. A view from each campsite is part of the spacious feeling that qualifies a campground for five stars in this category.

QUIET

Quiet is part of beautiful. There's nothing like the sound of a generator to ruin an otherwise exquisite campsite. I consider white noise, such as the roar of a river, to improve the quiet rating because it is natural and drowns out the sounds of other campers.

SECURITY

Most of the campsites in this guide have campground hosts who keep a good eye on the property, which makes the campground safer than a good neighborhood. The farther the campground is from an urban center, the more secure it is. Of course, you can leave your valuables with the hosts if you're going to be gone for a day or so, but don't leave little things lying around. A blue jay will take off with a pair of sunglasses, and you never can tell what a visiting bear will decide has food value.

CLEANLINESS

Most campgrounds in this guide are well tended. Sometimes, on big weekends, places can get a little rank—not unlike one's kitchen after a big party. I appreciate the little things like the campground host who came around with a rake after each site was vacated to police the place. That particular campground received five stars in the cleanliness department.

THE CAMPGROUND PROFILE

Each profile contains a concise but informative narrative that describes the campground and individual sites. Readers get a sense not only of the property itself but also the recreational opportunities available nearby. This descriptive text is enhanced with three helpful sidebars: Ratings, Key Information, and Getting There (accurate driving directions that lead you to the campground from the nearest major roadway).

THE CAMPGROUND LOCATOR MAP AND MAP LEGEND

Use the Southern California Campground Locator Map on page iv to assess the exact location of each campground. The campground's number appears not only on the overview map but also in the table of contents and on the profile's first page.

A map legend that details the symbols found on the campground-layout maps appears immediately following the table of contents, on page vii.

CAMPGROUND-LAYOUT MAPS

Each profile includes a detailed map of individual campsites, roads, facilities, and other key elements.

GPS CAMPGROUND-ENTRANCE COORDINATES

Readers can easily access all campgrounds in this book by using the directions given and the overview map, which shows at least one major road leading into the area. But for those who enjoy using GPS technology to navigate, the book includes coordinates for each campground's entrance in latitude and longitude, expressed in degrees, minutes, and seconds.

To convert GPS coordinates from degrees and decimal minutes and decimal degrees to the above degrees, minutes, and seconds format, use one of the many online tools for converting coordinates. For more on GPS technology, visit usgs.gov.

A note of caution: A dedicated GPS unit will easily guide you to any of these campgrounds, but users of smartphone mapping apps may find that cell service is often unavailable in the remote areas where many of these hideaways are located.

ABOUT THIS BOOK

Drive from a campground below sea level in Death Valley to a campground 10,000 feet up by a glacier in the Sierras in two hours. This diversity is Southern California camping. The Big Sur coast is a wonder of the world. Anza-Borrego Desert State Park is as big as Rhode Island. In the southern mountains, Mount San Jacinto feels like little Switzerland. Near Julian, you'd swear you were in Vermont. The beaches of the southern coast are legendary.

GEOGRAPHY

For the purposes of this book, Southern California is everything below a line drawn from Santa Cruz across the top of Yosemite National Park to the Nevada border. This area is divided into the Coast, the Desert, the Northern Sierras, and the Southern Sierras.

These four areas represent an amazing diversity in terrain. The Coast includes the 200 miles of sandy beaches north of the Mexican border to above Santa Barbara, and the mountains that parallel the shore above the Los Angeles Basin to Santa Cruz. The Desert, in the southeast corner of California, is a vast and fascinating area of three deserts—Mojave, Colorado, and Sonoran—extending to the Colorado River. The Northern Sierras, or Sierra Nevada, the largest mountain mass in the United States, extends north from the Mojave Desert to Sequoia, Kings Canyon, and Yosemite. The Southern Sierras include the San Bernardinos and other minor ranges that extend southeast into Mexico.

WHERE TO GO AND WHEN

Pleasant camping can be found on the coast year-round. For winter and early spring camping, head for the desert. Between Death Valley National Park, East Mojave National Preserve, Joshua Tree National Park, and Anza-Borrego Desert State Park you could camp all winter and never stay in the same spot twice. Camp in the Northern and Southern Sierras in the spring, summer, and fall. The southern beaches are a year-round affair. Never camp in the desert in summer, and only camp in the mountains in the winter if you are prepared to go snow camping.

WEATHER

When a guidebook covers an area of such environmental diversity, it's tough to sum up what kind of weather visitors should expect. However, if one word can be used to describe the overall weather of the southern half of California, it would be *arid*. Though this diverse environment will bring heat, rain, snow, hail, wind, and freezing cold temps, you're unlikely to experience real humidity, only days that are relatively muggy. That said, you should always be prepared. Read weather reports and never assume you won't need rain gear or warm undergarments and layers. In higher elevations, almost anything can happen at any time. In coastal areas, it can be unexpectedly chilly and cloudy well into early summer. In desert areas, temps can drop below freezing at night and rise into the 90s in the day. Never, ever underestimate the heat. There are places in this guidebook that regularly see temps in the 100-plus range.

ANIMAL AND PLANT HAZARDS

A wide range of plants and animals in Southern California can potentially hurt you, but only a few actually pose a significant threat. By far, the most dangerous is Toxicodendron diversilobum, or **Western poison oak** (see photo at right). This nasty shrub affects more people's lives than any other living thing in the state. If you touch it, an itchy, blistery rash could result. Memorize what it looks like and avoid it at all costs. It's mostly found in shaded areas, from sea level to 5,000 feet. In fall, when its signature three-leaf adornments have dried and fallen off, this plant is dangerous—the stems are as infectious, if not more so, than the leaves.

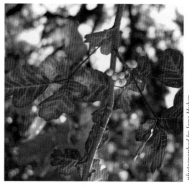

photographed by Jane Huber

The next most dangerous living thing (to humans) is the **rattlesnake**. There are numerous species in this state, and they're all potentially lethal. The more common Northern Pacific and Southern Pacific rattlesnakes' fangs inject a nasty hemotoxic venom, which essentially destroys bodily tissue. This is why amputations are common in victims. The Northern Mohave rattlesnake is even worse—its venom is also neurotoxic, meaning it can cause paralysis. The best way to avoid being bitten by rattlesnakes is to avoid stepping or sitting on them. This may seem self-explanatory, but if you find yourself in any situation where you can't see where you're sitting or stepping (during night hikes or bushwhacking expeditions), you're asking for trouble. If the unthinkable happens, seek medical attention IMMEDIATELY. Antivenin is the only remedy for a snakebite, so drop everything and get to the nearest hospital, or call 911.

Black bears and **mountain lions** are a distant third and fourth, respectively, in terms of danger. Black bears are seen quite frequently in higher elevations and will usually spook and retreat once they see you. They're drawn to food, so keep your campsites neat, store your food in a bear-proof receptacle if possible, and most likely you'll be fine. Attacks are extremely rare, but if one occurs, do not play dead (as you would in a grizzly or brown bear attack); fight as hard as you can and try to escape. Mountain lion attacks are so rare they're almost not worth mentioning. Like black bears, mountain lions usually don't want any trouble and will retreat as soon as they see you. However, if you do find yourself staring down one of these giant felines in close quarters, don't run. Make yourself look big as possible and back away slowly, maintaining eye contact. If one attacks, fight back with all your might.

FIRST AID KIT

A useful first aid kit may contain more items than you might think necessary. These are just the basics. Prepackaged kits in waterproof bags (Atwater Carey and Adventure Medical make them) are available. As a preventive measure, take along sunscreen and bug spray. Even though quite a few items are listed here, they pack down into a small space:

- Ace bandages or Spenco joint wraps
- Adhesive bandages, such as Band-Aids
- Antibiotic ointment (Neosporin or the generic equivalent)
- Antiseptic or disinfectant, such as Betadine or hydrogen peroxide
- Aspirin, acetaminophen (Tylenol), or ibuprofen (Advil)
- Benadryl or the generic equivalent, diphenhydramine (in case of allergic reactions)
- Butterfly-closure bandages
- Comb and tweezers (for removing ticks from your skin)
- Epinephrine in a prefilled syringe (for severe allergic reactions to outdoor mishaps such as bee stings)
- Gauze (one roll and six 4-by-4-inch compress pads)
- LED flashlight or headlamp
- Matches or lighter
- Moist towlettes
- Moleskin/Spenco 2nd Skin
- Pocketknife or multipurpose tool
- Waterproof first aid tape
- Whistle (for signaling rescuers if you get lost or hurt)

GOOD PLANNING

A little planning makes a good camping trip great. First, decide where and when you want to go. Then, phone that district's ranger headquarters to make sure the campground is open and that it has water. See if the ranger recommends other campgrounds. Ask if it's going to be busy. If it is, reserve ahead if possible. All national forest campgrounds must be reserved at least three to seven days in advance. (Note: For all reservable campgrounds in this book, there is an $8 fee if you book through reserveamerica.com or a $9–$10 fee if you reserve through recreation.gov.) Remember, if you arrive and don't like the reserved site, the campground host will move you if another site is available.

Next, get your equipment together. Everybody knows what basics to bring tent camping. A tent (of course), the sleeping bags, a cooler, a stove, pots, utensils, a water jug, matches, a can opener, etc. But, it's those little things that you suddenly wish you had that make a happy camper.

- **BRING EARPLUGS.** You might need earplugs to get a good snooze. The first night or two out camping, the unfamiliar flap of the tent fabric might drive you crazy if you don't have earplugs. Also, a snoring mate sleeping a foot away from you is nighttime hell on earth without earplugs.

- **DON'T FORGET TO PACK YOUR OWN PILLOW.** A good pillow gets your shoulders off the deck and lets your hips and behind take the weight. Use your clothes bag as an additional pillow (also consider inflatable pillows sold at camping stores).

- **BRING A THIN FOAM MATTRESS OR SELF-INFLATING PAD.** Buy a spider-mat, a device that keeps your pad from slipping on the tent floor and keeps your sleeping bag on top of it. Air mattresses are OK but susceptible to puncture. Never buy a double air mattress—every time your mate moves you get tossed around. Get a sleeping bag that is good and warm. Nothing is worse than being cold at night, and no sleeping bag is too warm. Bring a sheet so you can sleep under it at first, then crawl into the bag when it gets nippy.

- **CHECK THE WEATHER.** If it's going to be cold, remember to bring socks and sweatpants to sleep in. A sweatshirt with a hood is invaluable, since you lose a lot of heat through your head.

- **BRING A WATER BOTTLE FROM WHICH TO DRINK AT NIGHT.** Consequently, a pee jar (a pee pot for ladies) just outside the tent is a great idea. You can stumble outside, use it, and empty it in the toilet in the morning.

- **BRING SOMETHING TO PUT OUTSIDE THE TENT TO CLEAN YOUR FEET ON.** In the woods, a square of AstroTurf works fine. At the seashore or in the desert, a tray full of water in which to dip your feet works best. Bring a small brush for what grit leaks in.

- **REMEMBER FLASHLIGHTS.** The little mini-mags work OK, and if you take off the lens, you can hang them from a tent loop and actually read. Be careful since the little bulb is hot and will burn fabric or fingers. What works even better is a headlamp. Just strap the lamp around your head with an adjustable elastic band. Everywhere you look, there's light. They're great for finding stuff, cleaning up in the dark after dinner, and reading.

- **BRING DUCT TAPE.** "If you can't fix it, duct-tape it" is a camping maxim.

- **BRING A SPONGE TO CLEAN OFF THE PICNIC TABLE.** A plastic tablecloth is nice, too (bring little pushpins to secure it so it won't blow away). A plastic bowl or a Sea to Summit Kitchen Sink from REI (rei.com) can be invaluable for washing dishes. Picnic table benches get mighty hard, so bring a cushion.

- **BUY A CHEAP LAWN CHAIR** and get the inexpensive umbrella that attaches to the back of the chair, so you can sit around camp out of the sun.

- **BRING A LITTLE LEAF RAKE** to police your camp area.

- **REMEMBER BINOCULARS, A BIRD BOOK, AND A WILDFLOWER BOOK,** so you can put a name with what you see.

- **DON'T BE AFRAID TO ASK FELLOW CAMPERS FOR HELP** or for stuff you might have forgotten. All campers know what it's like to forget basic stuff and many love to help fellow campers. There might be a vacationing mechanic camping in the next site over when your car won't start or somebody with extra white gas for your stove. Be friendly to your fellow campers. Wave and say hi.

- **THE CAMPFIRE IS AN IMPORTANT CAMP EVENT.** Stores around the campground sell bundles of wood and, often, the campground host and hostess sell wood. Also, there may be windfalls around the campground from which you can take wood (ask the campground host). You need a good camp saw for that. An absolute essential is a can of charcoal starter fluid. This guarantees a fire even in a driving rain. Naturally, don't forget marshmallows, graham crackers, and chocolate for roasting.

- **CHECK YOUR CAR BEFORE YOU GO.** A mechanical breakdown on your way is a big bummer. Have a mechanic check your water hoses and the air pressure in your tires before you load up. Remember, your car will be loaded down with stuff, and this will put a strain on your tires and cooling system. Bring an extra fan belt. Nothing can shut down the car like a snapped fan belt that you have to special order from Japan. Even if you don't know a fan belt from third base, bring one. Somebody will come along who knows how to install it. Make sure your spare tire is correctly inflated. Mishap #999 is when you put on your spare, let the car down, and find out the spare is flat.

- **IF YOU FISH, BE SURE TO GET A LICENSE AND DISPLAY IT.** Fishing without a license is a misdemeanor, punishable by a maximum fine of $1,000 and/or six months in jail. On your way into the campground, stop at a local store and find out what the folks are using for bait. Buy it. This will save you a lot of experimentation and probably provide you with a good meal.

- **REMEMBER THE BEARS!** Never leave your cooler out. Put it in the trunk or disguise it with a blanket if you have a hatchback or a van. Don't eat in your tent. Take all cosmetics, soap, etc. and put them in the car. Disguise them too. A bear will rip off a car door to get a tube of lip balm. Bring a small bottle of bleach to wipe down your picnic table at night—bears don't like bleach (but don't put too much faith in this!). If a bear raids your camp looking for food, shoo him away like you would a naughty dog. Don't worry. Even the boldest black bears don't go into tents unless they smell food.

- **CONSIDER DISPERSED CAMPING.** With a fire permit, a shovel, and a bucket of water, you can camp just about anywhere in the national forests (consult ranger district headquarters) and in Anza-Borrego Desert State Park. The fire permit costs nothing, and there are miles and miles of fire roads and lumber roads you can explore to find the dispersed campground of your dreams.

SETTLING IN

When you come into a campground, be aware of a certain psychological barrier. This is a new place. Suddenly, you've driven all this way, and the campground doesn't look that hot. You feel disappointed. You feel like the "new kid at school." The other campers look up from their game of gin rummy and hope you won't camp next to them as you drive around the campground loops and look helplessly at the open sites. Nothing looks good enough.

Park your car. Pull into the first available site that could possibly do. Then, walk around the campground. You have half an hour to decide before you pick your site and pay. Once you get out and walk, you'll break through that "new kid at school" dilemma and soon feel like you're a part of the place. It's odd. Suddenly, you don't mind camping next to the gin rummy players. You realize that this is your campground as well as theirs. By the next morning, the whole place will feel like home, and the gin rummy players will seem like the best of neighbors. You won't understand why you didn't immediately recognize this campground as the best.

When you plan a camping trip, try to stay in one campground for at least three days. Stay one day, and you end up spending most of your time packing and unpacking and getting familiar with the campground. Stay three days, and you'll relax and have fun.

Go tent camping. Live in paradise for a few days. Camping makes you want to sin like the damned, sleep like the righteous, and hike like the last of the great American walkers. It's a balm for the weary soul!

THE COAST

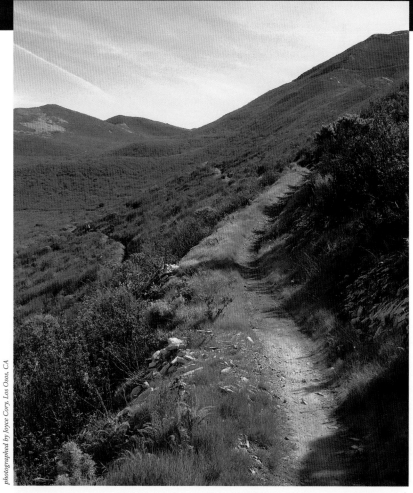

Mountain bikers enjoy the Beebe Trail in Montaña de Oro State Park (see page 31).

Catalina Island:
TWO HARBORS CAMPGROUND

Beauty ★★★★★ / Privacy ★★★ / Spaciousness ★★★★★ / Quiet ★★ / Security ★★★★ / Cleanliness ★★★★

A peaceful island paradise with crystal-blue waters, Catalina Island has miles of trails to hike and a plethora of aquatic activities.

Santa Catalina Island is one of seven islands located off the coast of Southern California. Although some are off-limits to visitors and difficult to access, Catalina Island is by far the most welcoming of this oft-overlooked island chain, with tent camping options galore. It's an unspoiled, unpolluted island waterfront camping utopia that gives visitors a chance to see what the California aquatic environment looked like before Western civilization settled here.

There's an assortment of great tent camping sites at Catalina Island, including hike-in and boat-in campsites. Two Harbors Campground requires neither extensive hiking to reach, nor a kayak, but you'll need to tackle an obvious problem—how to get to the island. The most affordable and popular way is by taking the Catalina Express shuttle to the island, from San Pedro. It's a short trip, under 1 hour, and the ticket prices are moderately priced at around $70 for a round-trip.

Weather is predictable at Catalina Island, and much like the weather anywhere on the California Coastline. The only wild card to be aware of is the super-annoying "June Gloom" or "May Gray." Correctly termed a marine layer, this meteorological curse is a layer of high fog that can last all day long—all weekend long, in fact. It happens randomly anytime in the late spring/early summer. It's not a deal-breaker, but it can be a buzzkill for scuba divers and

A view of Isthmus Harbor, looking west from above the campsites

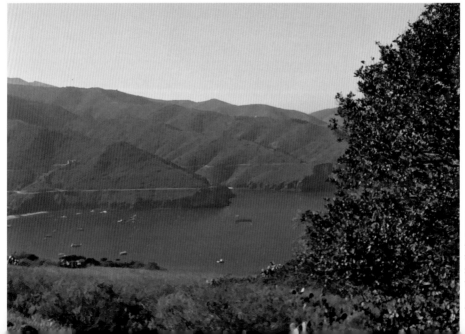

KEY INFORMATION

LOCATION: Two Harbors, Catalina Island, CA, 90704

CONTACT: 877-778-8322, visitcatalinaisland.com

OPERATED BY: Catalina Island Conservancy

OPEN: Year-round

SITES: 42

EACH SITE: Picnic table, fire ring

ASSIGNMENT: Reservations can be made at reserveamerica.com or 877-778-1487

REGISTRATION: Upon arrival, check in at Two Harbors Visitor Services, located on the dock in the center of town

PARKING: N/A

FACILITIES: Toilets, running water, cold water outdoor showers, pay-showers with hot water in town

FEE: Per-person, per day; adults: $25 (winter), $27 (summer), $28 (holidays); children: $16, $18, and $19, respectively

ELEVATION: Sea level

RESTRICTIONS:

PETS: Prohibited

FIRES: Permitted inside established fire rings

ALCOHOL: No restrictions

---

snorkelers, or anyone who digs sunshine and heat—the marine layer can drop temperatures to the low 70s when it's 100+ everywhere else. Rest assured, northerly winds will usually blow away this dreaded fog blanket by midafternoon. Or, book your trip in September or October, when the marine layer has packed up and left for the year.

For those who'd like to know where the name Two Harbors comes from, the area is situated on a narrow strip of land, or isthmus, between two natural bays on either side of the island—Isthmus Harbor on the north side, where the campground is located, and Catalina Harbor on the south side. Catalina Harbor—or Cat Harbor, as the locals call it—is a 0.5-mile walk from the arrival dock. It's a must see, but you'll probably need to set up camp first.

After you've disembarked from the Catalina Express shuttle and checked in, getting to the sites, which are situated along the shore at the east side of the bay, is a 0.25-mile walk with one steep hill to ascend. Thankfully, you'll be spared from schlepping your gear if you can pony up $5 to have the Two Harbors staff haul it to your site. Cool, right? The actual sites are carved into the bluffs above the shoreline. Each uniquely different site earns marks or demerits for privacy, views, coziness, proximity to shore, and general charm. Hopefully you've put Google Earth to use and have chosen wisely—this is a very popular place in the summer months. You can all but forget swapping sites once you're there.

Once settled, you're free to do almost anything you can think of. The small town of Two Harbors can outfit you for scuba diving, snorkeling, stand-up paddleboarding, mountain biking, kayaking, and more. Fishing, spearfishing, and gathering lobsters are allowed, provided you're licensed and abide by strictly enforced California Department of Fish and Wildlife regulations (learn more online at wildlife.ca.gov). Don't forget hiking; there are hundreds of miles of singletrack trails and fire roads to explore. However, if there's one activity you shouldn't miss, it's snorkeling. The water clarity is incredible inside Isthmus Harbor, especially in the late summer. There's lots of aquatic life to see, especially if you swim around the rocky point to the east or to the harbor reef, marked with tower and navigation light in the middle of the bay. In winter, spring, and fall, the diving is great, but the water will chill you to the bone, so bring a wet suit.

When the sun drops beneath the horizon, unless it's an unusually dry season you're free to make campfires inside fire rings, with firewood that can be delivered from the general store in town. If you're feeling social, Harbor Reef Restaurant has a full bar and live music on occasion. Things can get really silly down there, especially during the infamous Buccaneer Days festival. Happening on the first weekend of October, it's a three-day, pirate-themed island bender, with live-music, multiple bars, costume contests, treasure hunts, and lots of booze. If interested, plan early—the campsites will be 100% reserved as much as a year in advance.

Chances are, those pesky hoops you had to jump through to get to Two Harbors will be all but forgotten when you board the Catalina Express boat and head back to San Pedro. There's nothing like it. It very well could be the ultimate Los Angeles staycation. You might not guess it, but the entirety of the island lies inside Los Angeles County.

Catalina Island: Two Harbors Campground

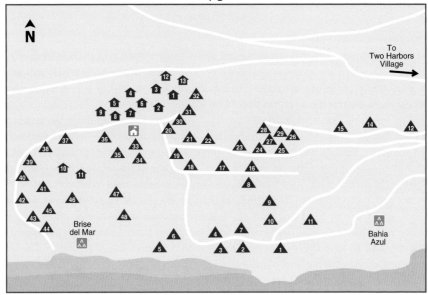

GETTING THERE

The Catalina Sea and Air Terminal is located at Berth 95, San Pedro, CA 90731. To get there, from anywhere, make your way to the I-110 Harbor Freeway and head southbound toward San Pedro. Take exit 1A, drive to Swinford Street, and continue until you arrive at the Catalina Sea and Air Terminal.

GPS COORDINATES
CATALINA SEA AND AIR TERMINAL: N33° 44' 56.2" W118° 16' 28"
TWO HARBORS: N33° 26' 25" W118° 29' 31"

El Capitán State Beach Campground

Beauty ★★★★★ / Privacy ★★★ / Spaciousness ★★★★ / Quiet ★★★ / Security ★★★ / Cleanliness ★★★★

Many SoCal locals believe El Capitán is by far the ultimate campground in California.

Though not quite the place to seek pure tent camping solitude, El Capitán State Beach may be the ultimate slice of unspoiled California beach heaven. This massive camping facility, located on a bluff above the beach, is the prime locale for every beach activity imaginable: sunbathing, surfing, kayaking, stand-up paddleboarding, and more. Although the camping area is often bustling with visitors and large RVs, you can easily find peace and quiet when you need it. There are acres of prime beach real estate below, perfect for all-day lounging sessions—just don't forget your cooler, umbrella, and sunblock.

The attraction of El Capitán has everything to do with its geography. The campsites are perched in a grove of oak trees atop a bluff above the shoreline. Most sites have unobstructed ocean views, and many offer natural privacy. Although there are no sites on the sandy beach itself, several easy-to-find trails lead down to various sections of shoreline. El Capitán State Beach lies on a point, and surfers will love the point break to the east of the sites when the swells are up. During low tides, tidepools will appear around the east end of the point for beach walkers to explore.

There are always a few among us who don't particularly enjoy the ocean—but they needn't stay home, because there's a great bike path that runs for 2 miles, connecting El

Surfers, hikers, and bird-watchers share the beach.

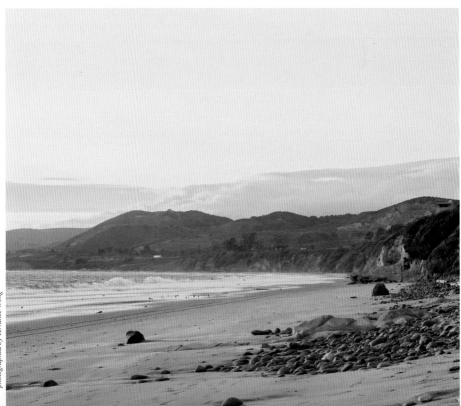

KEY INFORMATION

LOCATION: 2 El Capitán State Beach Road, Goleta, CA 93117

CONTACT: 805-968-1033, parks.ca.gov

OPERATED BY: California State Parks

OPEN: Year-round

SITES: 132

EACH SITE: Picnic table, fire ring

ASSIGNMENT: First come, first served December 1–March 31; other months allow reservations at reservecalifornia.com or 800-444-7275

REGISTRATION: Self-registration if park entrance station is closed

FACILITIES: Bathrooms, running water, pay showers (25¢ for 2 minutes)

PARKING: At site

FEE: $45 plus $8 nonrefundable reservation fee

ELEVATION: Sea level

RESTRICTIONS:

PETS: Dogs must be kept on a 6-foot leash at all times, are not permitted on the beach or in buildings, and must be inside vehicle or tent at night.

FIRES: Permitted within established fire rings

ALCOHOL: No restrictions

Capitán State Beach with Refugio State Beach. The path allows beachgoers easy access to the entire length of shoreline between the two parks. When you've grown weary of the sun and the sand, explore the hiking trails of the nearby El Capitán Canyon, located to the north, on the other side of US 101.

The ample shade among the campsites makes the beach camping manageable for people who are sensitive to the sun. Those who've spent all day under the sun understand this—it's

Sunset at El Capitán State Beach

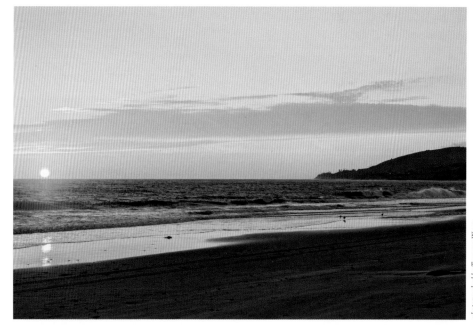

very easy to become overwhelmed with sun-spawned beach fatigue and get thoroughly "beached out." El Capitán allows visitors to fully escape the beach environment in the oak groves. Inside several sites it's quite possible to forget the beach entirely, because the immediate surroundings look like the typical chaparral environment of the interior.

Wildlife lovers should keep their eyes on water. In any season it's possible to see a variety of aquatic mammals, including dolphins, porpoise, gray whales, humpbacks, blue whales, and more. Fishermen and women will find themselves equally at home—shore fishing is permitted for licensed, regulation-abiding anglers, and the waters are fertile with several species of near-shore game fish.

Perhaps the icing on the cake for El Capitán is its relative solitude—the noise of the highway (US 101) is mitigated by the lapping surf below, although you will hear the sounds of passing trains occasionally. El Capitán truly is the "captain" of SoCal's state beach campgrounds, but with its pleasures comes a catch—there's a six-month waiting period for reservations.

El Capitán State Beach Campground

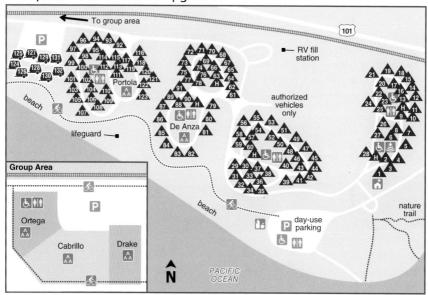

GETTING THERE

El Capitán State Beach is hard to miss—it's located 17 miles northwest of Santa Barbara off US 101, clearly marked with large signs.

GPS COORDINATES: N34° 27' 37" W120° 01' 26"

Fremont Peak State Park Campgrounds

Beauty ★★★★★ / Privacy ★★★ / Spaciousness ★★★★ / Quiet ★★★★ / Security ★★★ / Cleanliness ★★★

Come to Fremont Peak State Park for spring camping and to San Juan Bautista for California's days of yesteryear.

Fremont Peak State Park is deliriously pretty in April and May, when the spring grasses are green and feathery and the flowers are blooming. It's a great place to go when the coast is socked in with fog. Climb to the peak and look out over some of the richest farmland and marine areas in the world.

The drive up to the park from San Juan Bautista is alternately lovely, chilling, and lovely again. At first, you take a winding, old country road out of the valley and go up into oaks draped with mistletoe. Then you burst into *Road Warrior* country. On the left is the Hollister Hills State Vehicular Recreation Area, where off-road enthusiasts bring their vehicles. It's a land of tire-ripped hills and torched brush. Scary. But persevere and you will arrive at the mountaintop to enter Fremont Peak State Park, with its oaks, pines, and incredible views.

The camping here is primitive and best suited for tents. All the sites are roomy, grassy, and shaded by oaks. There is potable water, and each site boasts an incredible view of Monterey Bay. However, it is best to avoid the area in the summer, when Gavilan Peak is overrun by nasty little biting flies.

The park's namesake oversees vistas of Monterey Bay and the San Benito and Salinas Valleys.

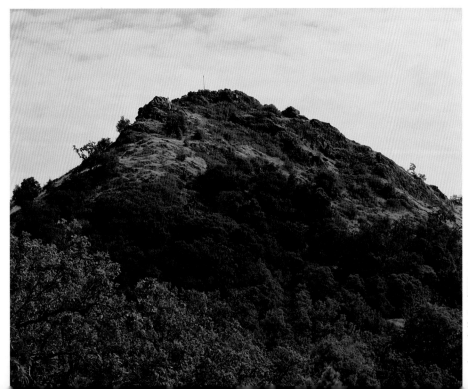

photographed by Daniel W. Hartwig

KEY INFORMATION

LOCATION: 10700 San Juan Canyon Road, San Juan Bautista, CA 95045

CONTACT: 831-623-4255, parks.ca.gov

OPERATED BY: California State Parks

OPEN: Year-round

SITES: 25

EACH SITE: Picnic table, fire ring

ASSIGNMENT: First come, first served or by reservation

REGISTRATION: At entrance or reserve at reservecalifornia.com or 800-444-7275

FACILITIES: Water, pit toilets, wheelchair-accessible sites

PARKING: At site

FEE: $25 plus $8 nonrefundable reservation fee

ELEVATION: 2,750'

RESTRICTIONS:

PETS: On leash in campgrounds only (not allowed on trails)

FIRES: In fire rings (no firewood available at campgrounds)

ALCOHOL: No restrictions

VEHICLES: Trailers up to 18 feet, RVs up to 26 feet

OTHER: Keep food stored in vehicle when not in campsite to prevent feral pig depredation.

Fremont Peak State Park is actually not situated on Fremont Peak, but on Gavilan Peak. The expansive view from Gavilan prompted John C. Frémont to build a fort there one fateful day in 1846. California, then a territory of Mexico, was seething. The Mexican government wanted to get rid of the American settlers, who were forming ragtag armies to take over the territory. In addition, American Indians were arming themselves and trying to retake their former lands. Into the middle of this rode John C. Frémont, a captain of the Corps of Topographical Engineers, to map the California Trail.

José Castro, the Mexican governor of California, ordered Frémont and his group of Delaware tribe members and hard-bitten frontiersmen to leave the territory. Frémont refused. Cheekily, he marched his men up Gavilan Peak and built a rough log fort within plain sight of General Castro's headquarters in San Juan Bautista. When Frémont raised the American flag up a stripped sapling, his men cheered, but General Castro was livid. He posted a proclamation:

Fellow Citizens: A band of robbers commanded by a captain of the United States Army, J. C. Frémont, have without respect to the laws and authorities of the department daringly introduced themselves into the country and disobeyed the orders both of your commander-in-chief and of the prefect of the district.

Castro summoned a band of Mexican cavalrymen from Monterey to head north to San Juan Bautista.

Frémont set an ambush for the cavalrymen, but at the last minute, the Mexican officers inexplicably ordered their troops back to Monterey. Meanwhile, on the peak, the westerly wind kicked up and blew the crude flagpole down. Taking this as a sign, Fremont abandoned his fort and grudgingly retreated.

General Castro called the Americans "cowards and poor guests," and the incident was over, but both Frémont and Castro would play giant roles in the subsequent turnover of Mexican California to the United States.

Located near the campgrounds, the Fremont Peak Observatory houses a 30-inch reflecting telescope. They have special programs in the spring and fall. For more information, including a schedule, visit fpoa.net or call 831-623-2465.

A good hike to the peak begins in the parking lot. You'll see a road and a trail. The trail, signed with a hiker's symbol, leads to the observatory. Take the road for a short distance, then join the signed Peak Trail, which circles the mountain.

On the high ridges, see Coulter pine and madrone. The northern slopes are full of manzanita, toyon, and scrub oak, and the southern slopes spill over with grasses and wildflowers. Don't forget your binoculars.

Visit San Juan Bautista, once the district headquarters of the northern half of Alta, California. The Great 1906 San Francisco earthquake destroyed half the town, and soon cows grazed on the plaza. As Will Durant once said, "Civilization exists by geological consent, subject to change without notice." San Juan slept until it was resurrected by benefactors of the Old Mission and the California Department of Parks and Recreation. I can't count the number of times I have driven US 101 and passed by San Juan Bautista. However, after one visit, I'm a believer. The Old Mission and the plaza have been lovingly restored.

Fremont Peak State Park Campgrounds

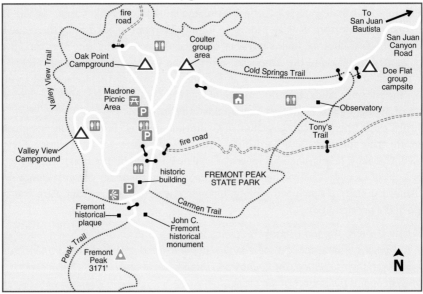

GETTING THERE

From Los Angeles, drive 330 miles north on US 101 to Salinas, then continue north on US 101 about 17 miles and turn east onto CA 156. Turn right (south) onto San Juan Canyon Road and drive 11 miles to the campgrounds along a narrow, winding road.

GPS COORDINATES: N35° 59' 24" W121° 29' 46"

Kirk Creek and Plaskett Creek Campgrounds

Beauty ★★★★★ / Privacy ★★★★★ / Spaciousness ★★★★★ / Quiet ★★★★★ / Security ★★★ / Cleanliness ★★★★★

Come for the huge cliffs of jade. Stay for great camping and hiking in the mountains.

Kirk Creek and Plaskett Creek Campgrounds are like fraternal twins. They occupy the most isolated stretch of CA 1, north of San Simeon and south of Big Sur. About 5 miles apart, on the best stretch of Los Padres National Forest coastline, these campgrounds offer the most relaxed camping on the entire Southern California coast.

Kirk Creek lies on a bluff overlooking the ocean. Set in gorse—a spiny, yellow-flowered bush—it gets quite a lot of wind. Of course, the view is shockingly immediate, as if you are suspended over the ocean itself. The sites are separated and private until you stand up; the brush surrounding the sites is about chest high. This does, however, give you some relief from the oceanic blasts. Thankfully, there's a fence along the edge of the precipice. Just south, goat trails lead down to a rocky point and a sandy cove at low tide. Navigate these trails during daylight hours.

Plaskett Creek Campground is designed for small RVs, with larger and more level sites. Plaskett is farther away from the beach, behind a line of Monterey pines, and not as subject to the ocean's gusty blasts. The area is nice and grassy. The sites are roomier, but not as private without the impenetrable gorse cover of Kirk.

I love both campgrounds. Many CA 1 tourists speed through this area, because you feel as if you're between the devil and the deep blue sea here.

Admire the rugged beauty of the Big Sur coastline.

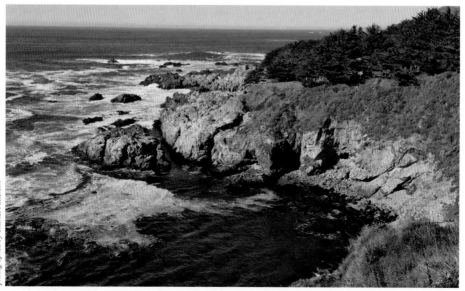

photographed by Charles Patterson

KEY INFORMATION

LOCATION: Kirk Creek: 64955 CA 1, Big Sur, CA 93920; Plaskett Creek: 69345 CA 1, Big Sur, CA 93920

CONTACT: 805-968-6640, www.fs.usda.gov/lpnf

OPERATED BY: U.S. Forest Service

OPEN: Year-round

SITES: Kirk 32, Plaskett 42

EACH SITE: Picnic table, fire ring

ASSIGNMENT: By reservation only (3 or more days in advance) at recreation.gov or 877-444-6777

REGISTRATION: At entrance

FACILITIES: Water, flush toilets

PARKING: At site

FEE: $35 plus $9 nonrefundable reservation fee

ELEVATION: Near sea level

RESTRICTIONS:

PETS: On leash only

FIRES: In fire pits

ALCOHOL: No restrictions

VEHICLES: Small RVs

OTHERS: 14-day stay limit

The nearby U.S. Forest Service station at Pacific Valley is primarily used as a fire station. An area map and other information are posted outside the station. The station does not have regularly scheduled hours of operation, but when personnel are on duty they are available to assist visitors. Maps are for sale.

There is hiking in the mountains directly east of the campground. Though the hiking is good and the weather is cool, the big draw here is the beach. Go to aptly named Jade Cove to see the huge cliffs made entirely of jade. What a magical experience! Walk down from the picnic area, over the cattle gate to the beach, and as the stairs hit the sand, you'll see the jade on the left. Then, continue south on the beach.

For another ocean experience, go pebble-hunting on the San Simeon coast. Find jadite and brown-and-green chert pebbles. American Indians fashioned arrowheads from chert. The best hunting is on Moonstone Beach. Turn off CA 1 in Cambria at Windsor Boulevard, then go northwest about 0.4 mile on Moonstone Beach Drive to the state beach parking area. Go down to the beach and walk northwest to the cliff. Also, try the beach at Pico Creek, 2.5 miles north of San Simeon Beach Campground.

GETTING THERE

From San Francisco, drive south on CA 1 through Monterey to Lucia. Then drive 4 miles farther south on CA 1 to Kirk Creek Campground on the right. Plaskett Creek Campground is 5.5 miles still farther south from Kirk Creek Campground. After you pass the ranger station, Plaskett Creek will be on your left.

Note: Due to road construction following landslide damage in Big Sur, CA 1 (Pacific Coast Highway) will be closed through summer 2018 and possibly longer at Mud Creek in the vicinity of Ragged Point. Please check dot.ca.gov for the latest road conditions, or visit maps.google.com to plan your alternate driving route.

GPS COORDINATES: N35° 59' 24" W121° 29' 46"

Kirk Creek Campground

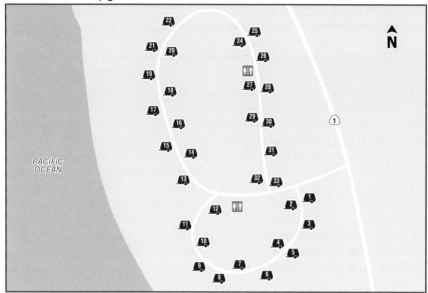

Plaskett Creek Campground

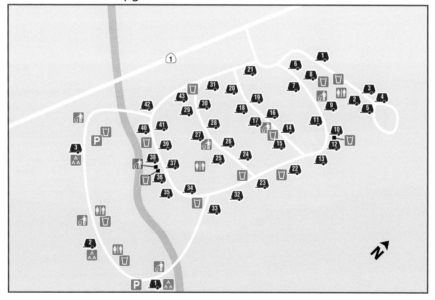

5

La Jolla Valley Hike-In Campground

Beauty ★★★★ / Privacy ★★★★★ / Spaciousness ★★★ / Quiet ★★★★★ / Security ★★★★★ / Cleanliness ★★★★★

The sites offer 360-degree views without any sign of civilization.

The La Jolla Valley Hike-In tent-camping sites are little known and seldom used. Little info about these campsites can be found anywhere, and you may not believe they exist until you motivate yourself to walk up there and take a look. A variety of routes lead to this destination, all of which offer picturesque views of the ocean amid pristine terrain. The number-one reason to visit this place: This is the only true backcountry campground in the Santa Monica Mountains. The sites offer 360-degree views without any sign of civilization, and you'll be hard-pressed to find another soul in the area.

For hikers, there are three logical routes to the La Jolla Valley area. With any of these routes, the objective is to reach La Jolla Valley Fire Road within the relatively small La Jolla Valley. Hikers coming from Ventura County may want to try the Chumash Trail, which leads directly to the campgrounds in a mostly northeasterly direction. Hikers from the Los Angeles area can make the trek via La Jolla Canyon Trail or by way of the Ray Miller Backbone Trail. La Jolla Canyon Trail leads almost directly to the sites, ending at La Jolla Valley Fire Road after roughly 2.5 miles, after which one would turn left and walk 0.3 mile, then look for the trails leading to the campgrounds on the right (north) side of the trail. Ray Miller Trail is the least direct, leading to a left turn on Overlook Trail followed by another

Solitude awaits in La Jolla Valley.

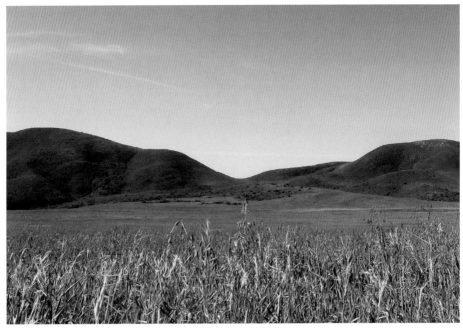

KEY INFORMATION

LOCATION: Ray Miller Trailhead off CA 1, Malibu, CA 90265

CONTACT: 818-880-0350, nps.gov/samo

OPERATED BY: California State Parks

OPEN: Year-round

SITES: 5

EACH SITE: Picnic table

ASSIGNMENT: First come, first served

REGISTRATION: Self-register by iron ranger at La Jolla Canyon park entrance

FACILITIES: Chemical toilets, no running water, trash must be packed out

PARKING: At La Jolla/Ray Miller parking area

FEE: $10 per person per night, auto-pay at the La Jolla/Ray Miller parking area

ELEVATION: 711'

RESTRICTIONS:

PETS: Prohibited

FIRES: Strictly prohibited

ALCOHOL: No restrictions

left on La Jolla Valley Fire Road, which leads to the campgrounds on the north side after 0.5 mile. Both routes are day hikes and suitable for hiking neophytes because the trails have no major technical challenges. It can be very hot, so it's essential to bring as much water as you can carry. Trail maps are available at the ranger kiosks of Big Sycamore Canyon and Thornhill Broome Beach.

You can also bike to La Jolla Valley if you enter via Big Sycamore Canyon-to-Overlook Trail (also referred to as Big Sycamore Canyon Loop Trail). This is highly recommended if you can carry camping gear on your mountain bike. Mountain biking is prohibited everywhere in La Jolla Valley except La Jolla Valley Fire Road, so walk your bike to the sites and stay off any singletracks in the area, no matter how much you're tempted.

Traveling to the sites may be the most appealing part of the tent-camping experience here. There's nothing like the peace and tranquility of Point Mugu State Park, and the refreshing sea breeze continually brought forth by the Pacific Ocean. This is prime Santa Monica Mountains chaparral scenery, so take it all in as you make the journey. Look for red-tailed hawks, bobcats, rattlesnakes, and deer along the way, and remember that your surroundings look much as they did when the earliest European explorers first came here.

It's impossible to visit these secluded sites and not wonder who frequented these areas before Europeans. The Chumash tribe made their home in the Santa Monica Mountains and other parts of Southern California. It's tough to imagine how they secured enough food to survive in such a dry, hot environment, and the answer lies within the oak acorn. The Chumash relied on the acorn as their vegetative staple, supplementing their diets with fish, sea mammals, birds, and land mammals, as well as other native plants. Because hunting in the Santa Monica Mountains is illegal, you'll have to survive on whatever food you packed in.

The trail that leads to the five tent sites (numbered 5–9) is a few steps west of the larger group camping sites. The entrance is marked with a small sign that reads LA JOLLA VALLEY TRAIL CAMP; it leads to a chemical toilet, beyond which are sites 5–9 on either side of a narrow trail heading in a northward direction. Along the trail are a few nonfunctional water spigots. There are no trash receptacles, so you'll have to carry everything out. This is a very special place, so it's especially important to follow the Leave No Trace principle here.

The sites feel very secluded because each has its own narrow, singletrack "driveway" leading to a space carved out of the dense foliage and containing one picnic table and just enough space for a tent or two. Due to the denseness of the vegetation, each site seems totally isolated because the other sites cannot be seen from any vantage point. You may see makeshift fire rings or evidence of campfires, but don't make a fire under any circumstances—you're surrounded by acres of dry, combustible tinder, and fires are strictly prohibited.

Once you've settled in, you can appreciate the peace and remoteness of the area. You may, in fact, be spooked by the wildness and seclusion. The La Jolla Valley hike-in campsites are for nature lovers who crave solitude and really want to get away. The experience isn't available anywhere else in the Santa Monica Mountains—it's definitely worthwhile.

La Jolla Valley Walk-In Campground

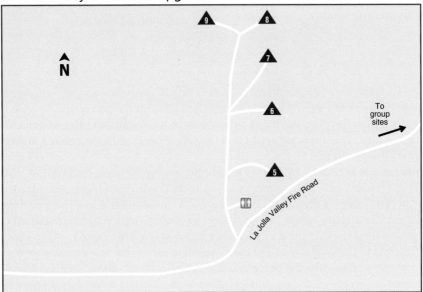

GETTING THERE

From Los Angeles, drive west on I-10 until it ends and becomes CA 1, or Pacific Coast Highway. Driving west, stay on CA 1 for 32.7 miles until you reach Big Sycamore Canyon Campground on the right, beyond Malibu. La Jolla Canyon Campground is 1.75 miles farther, also on the right.

GPS COORDINATES: N34° 06' 27" W119° 02' 10"

6

Leo Carrillo State Park Campground

Beauty ★★★★★ / Privacy ★★★ / Spaciousness ★★★★ / Quiet ★★★ / Security ★★★ / Cleanliness ★★★★★

After one visit to Leo Carrillo, you'll be hooked.

At first glance, Leo Carrillo State Park Campground looks similar to the nearby facility at Sycamore Canyon, but Leo Carrillo caters to a different clientele. While it lacks the world-class mountain-bike trails of Sycamore, the beach at Leo Carrillo State Park is the hot destination for aquatic pastimes like surfing, windsurfing, kite-surfing, scuba diving, sport fishing, stand-up paddleboarding, kayaking, and more. Leo Carrillo is prime ground for all of these pursuits, and even more.

Unlike Sycamore's main beach, Leo Carrillo's is protected by rocky obstructions that block the open ocean surge and provide safer waters for casual swimmers at the main beach. It's also a sunbather's paradise, with almost 2 miles of sparsely inhabited sandy beach to the south providing plenty of space for privacy and summertime bliss. The beach is highly picturesque and even offers an easily accessible sea cave. At low tide, amazing assortments of tidepools are exposed, giving the kids plenty to do.

Just as they do at Sycamore Canyon, campers access the beaches by walking through a creek-wash tunnel underneath the Pacific Coast Highway. Across the highway, 135 tent campsites are arrayed along the narrows of Arroyo Sequit Creek. The sites are spacious, and many offer natural borders and privacy with adequate separation between sites, along with plenty of shade provided by tall sycamore trees.

The area surrounding the campsites is a peaceful riparian landscape, much like Malibu's Surfrider Beach and Topanga Beach would have looked before urban development. Giving your skin a break with an afternoon nap under the shade of the sycamores is a highly

Explore the tidepools and reefs at Leo Carrillo State Park.

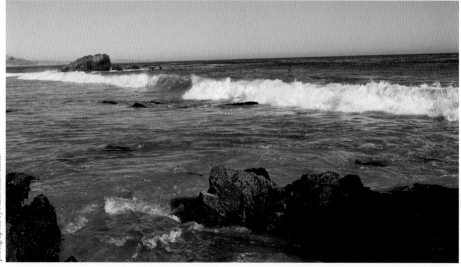

photographed by Maximilian Sluiter

KEY INFORMATION

LOCATION: 35000 West Pacific Coast Highway Malibu, CA 90265

CONTACT: 818-880-0363, parks.ca.gov

OPERATED BY: California State Parks

OPEN: Year-round

SITES: 135

EACH SITE: Picnic table, fire ring

ASSIGNMENT: First come, first served or by reservation

REGISTRATION: At park entrance or reserve at reservecalifornia.com or 800-444-7275

FACILITIES: Running water, bathrooms, showers, camp store

PARKING: $12

FEE: $45 plus $8 nonrefundable reservation fee

ELEVATION: Sea level

RESTRICTIONS:

PETS: Dogs must be kept on a 6-foot leash at all times, are not permitted on beach or in buildings, and must be inside vehicle or tent at night.

---

effective destressor. There are also great hiking trails to explore, including Yellow Hill and Nicholas Flat Trails.

Leo Carrillo State Park was named after Hollywood character actor Leo Carrillo (1880–1961), who played typecast roles for most of his career but was most remembered for his role as Pancho in the 1950s TV show *The Cisco Kid*. The beach wasn't, however, given his name to honor his contributions to entertainment: Carrillo was also an influential conservationist and preservationist. While serving on the California Beach and Parks Commission, Carrillo helped add Hearst Castle in San Simeon and Anza-Borrego Desert State Parks to California's inventory. His efforts are honored elsewhere in California: Leo Carrillo Elementary School in Westminster and Leo Carrillo Ranch Historic Park in Carlsbad. The Hollywood connection doesn't end with Carrillo; the beach named after him has been

Discover the coastal caves along the shore.

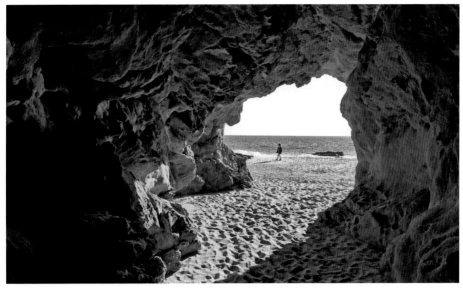

a popular locale for high-profile film and photographic shoots for many years, the most memorable being *Grease, The Karate Kid,* and *Point Break.*

Those unfamiliar with California beaches may find themselves startled by the chilliness of the water, even during the hottest months of the year. At its warmest, the waters off Leo Carrillo State Beach seldom exceed 65°F and drop to the mid-50s or lower during the winter and spring. Oceanic currents are to blame; the California Current sends a massive river of cold water southward along the Pacific Coast. Fittingly, amphibious folks will find themselves in wet suits frequently. Full-body suits are suitable for winter surfing; a 3-millimeter thickness will suffice. Free divers/snorkelers will do OK with the same gear but will probably also need neoprene hoods to stay warm. Scuba requires more drastic measures—7-millimeter suits, gloves, hoods, and booties are mandatory for most divers.

Camping at Leo Carrillo offers greatness in two environments—the beach and the wilderness. Understandably, there's a six-month waiting list for reservations during the peak season (March 1 to November 30). After one visit, you'll be addicted, possibly camping at Leo Carrillo every year, even if you're a local and thought you were jaded and somehow bored with SoCal's beaches. If a campsite can't be secured until the following summer, a day trip to this cherished locale is highly recommended and worth every penny spent on gasoline.

Leo Carrillo State Park Campground

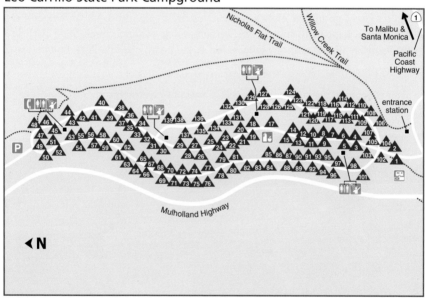

GETTING THERE

Leo Carrillo State Park is highly visible from the Pacific Coast Highway. From Santa Monica, head northwest on the Pacific Coast Highway for approximately 26.5 miles, after which Leo Carrillo State Park will appear on the right side of the road, clearly marked with signs. From Oxnard, look for Leo Carrillo State Beach after 16 miles on the Pacific Coast Highway heading southeast.

GPS COORDINATES: N34° 05' 53" W118° 56' 01"

7

Malibu Creek State Park Campground

Beauty ★★★★★ / Privacy ★ / Spaciousness ★★ / Quiet ★★★ / Security ★★★★★ / Cleanliness ★★★★

A good base camp from which to explore Los Angeles, the campground offers easy hiking and bicycling, and it's also good for kids.

Situated on a big hunk of the most coveted real estate in Southern California and surrounded by the rapidly encroaching megalopolis of the Los Angeles metropolitan area, Malibu Creek State Park Campground is a precious gem. With sections once owned by Bob Hope, Ronald Reagan, and 20th Century Fox, the park now covers more than 7,000 acres. This is a great place to tent camp in fall, winter, and spring. Protected by a mountain range from the springtime fog that hits the beaches in Southern California, Malibu Creek State Park is situated between two major tourist thoroughfares: CA 1 and US 101. It's just 40 miles down the hill to Malibu and all the wonderful beaches. You're also near Santa Barbara on US 101 and Universal City to the east.

You'll find safe mountain biking and hiking, so this is a great place to bring children camping. It's also a good first night's camp if you are flying into LAX, and a good escape from L.A. if you happen to live there. I've camped at Malibu Creek State Park several times on Saturday nights with my wife, eaten at the nearby Saddle Peak Lodge (excellent

Some of the park's trails offer a chance to experience the setting via horseback.

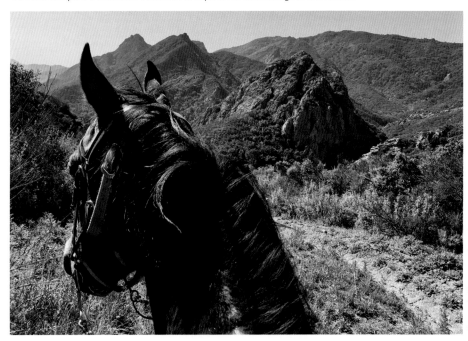

photographed by Kristina Bliss and Brave

KEY INFORMATION

LOCATION: 1925 Las Virgenes Road, Calabasas, CA 91302

CONTACT: 818-880-0367, parks.ca.gov

OPERATED BY: California State Parks

OPEN: Year-round

SITES: 63 tent sites; 4 RV sites

EACH SITE: Picnic table, fire ring, no hookups

ASSIGNMENT: First come, first served; reservations recommended in summer and on holidays

REGISTRATION: At park entrance or reserve at reservecalifornia.com or 800-444-7275

FACILITIES: Water, flush toilets, solar-heated showers (all accessible to disabled patrons)

PARKING: At site

FEE: $45 plus $8 nonrefundable reservation fee

ELEVATION: 500'

RESTRICTIONS:

PETS: On leash in campground only (not allowed on trails)

FIRES: Charcoal fires permitted year-round; wood fires may be restricted; check signs

ALCOHOL: No restrictions

VEHICLES: RVs up to 32 feet

OTHER: Be careful with fire.

---

food), then ducked back to our humble tent for a weekend combining the high life and the great outdoors.

High season at the campground begins with spring break and goes through the end of September. Since Malibu Creek can get crowded, be sure to come early on weekends during the summer. The ranger recommended arriving by noon on Friday to reserve a spot for a summer weekend. The campground is very clean, well patrolled, and well maintained, but the sites themselves are unremarkable. The incredible vista and the "neighborhood" are what make this a fun camping experience.

A good introductory walk is along Crags Road to Century Lake, then back again. From the campground, walk down to a wide fire road. Cross the stream, and you'll see that the road splits into a high road and a low road. Either one will do. Pass the visitor center and find the Gorge Trail. Follow it upstream to where the creek turns dramatically around volcanic rock cliffs into the Rock Pool. Remember the Tarzan movies and the *Swiss Family Robinson* TV series? Parts from both were filmed here.

Back on the high road, you'll come to the crest of a hill where you can look down on Century Lake. Look around carefully and spot the distinctive hills that doubled for Korean terrain in the TV series *M*A*S*H*.

A challenging hike is up to the Backbone Trail. From there, you could conceivably hike all the way to Will Rogers State Historic Park in Los Angeles. Don't try it, though, unless you are a walking fool. Farther on is a swampy pond always good for bird-watching, and then Ronald Reagan's ranch with some good hiking. (Obtain a good map of the park from the ranger at the gate for $1.)

For avid mountain bikers, this state park is an excellent staging area. If you're ambitious and fit enough, try climbing the infamous Bulldog Motorway. Simply head east on Crags Road thru the *M*A*S*H* site, then follow the signs from Bulldog Lateral to Bulldog Motorway, which are both left turns if heading eastward. After seemly endless switchbacks, Bulldog terminates at Castro Motorway. If you don't make it all the way, don't fret—this is a black-diamond ascent. From there, simply turn around and descend back to Malibu Creek, or explore farther. The Backbone multiuse trail is just a few pedal strokes away; just don't forget your GPS or trail map.

Note that wood fires are only conditionally allowed December–May because of summer fire hazards. This area is near the scene of the 1996 fire that burned down into the heart of Malibu Canyon, wreaking havoc on forests and homes. Fires in the Lower Chaparral are as common as cats and so much a part of the cycle of nature that American Indians would set controlled fires to help Mother Nature along. They were interested in burning the brush fuel underneath the bigger trees before the brush grew enough to burn the larger trees. Fire also allowed more access and helped expose the game animals.

My favorite time of year here is from fall to spring—the park's off-season. I find the mountains too hot in the summer for hiking or biking (pack a canteen if you decide to visit then). However, camping at Malibu Creek State Park in the summer would afford you a good base camp to hit the beach and other L.A. summer tourist attractions.

Malibu Creek State Park Campground

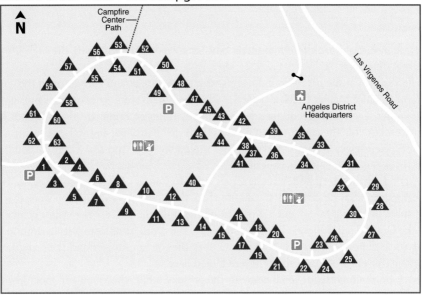

GETTING THERE

From Santa Monica, drive north up CA 1 through Malibu, turn right on Malibu Canyon Road, and drive 6 miles to the park entrance on the left. From the San Fernando Valley, drive north on US 101 to the Las Virgenes exit and drive 4 miles southwest on Las Virgenes Road to the park entrance.

GPS COORDINATES: N34° 5' 49" W118° 42' 51"

8

Montaña de Oro State Park:
ISLAY CREEK CAMPGROUND

Beauty ★★★★★ / Privacy ★★ / Spaciousness ★★★ / Quiet ★★ / Security ★★★★★ / Cleanliness ★★★★★

Here you can enjoy year-round camping with 7 miles of virgin California coast.

After a week, smoggy Los Angeles seems full of snarling attack dogs and urbanites ready to carve out your liver over a parking space. But drive north of Santa Barbara, where the air is clear, and you'll see hikers on cliffs at sunset, parents with babies in backpacks, ball-chasing Labrador retrievers, and unattended bicycles—especially at Montaña de Oro State Park. Its rocky azure coves feel like Greece; the sandwiched cliffs jutting out over the ocean are reminiscent of Cornwall; and the long sand dunes resemble Provincetown on Cape Cod. With 7 miles of spectacular coast, this is one of California's largest state parks.

Montaña de Oro was Chumash Indian territory until the Spanish Mission Period. The Chumash were missionized, then left without a way of life when the missions were secularized. Then came the Pechos, a Spanish family who dealt in cattle, and the ranching Spooners. Then Alexander Hazard planted hundreds of eucalyptus trees here in hopes of selling them to the railroad for ties. Hazard's lumber dreams hit the same rocks as those of other Southern California eucalyptus timber barons. The trees grew fast, but the tree grain spindled, making the tree useless—even as firewood.

Fiddle-necks adorn the Bluff Trail.

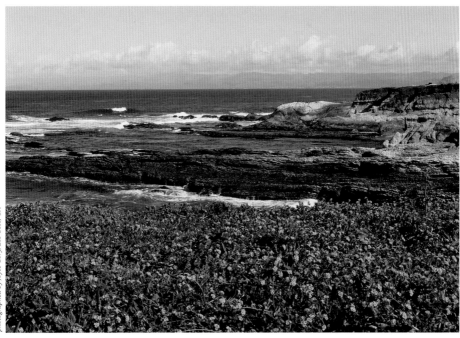

photographed by Joyce Cory, Los Osos, CA

KEY INFORMATION

LOCATION: 3550 Pecho Valley Road, Los Osos, CA 93402

CONTACT: 805-528-0513, parks.ca.gov

OPERATED BY: California State Parks

OPEN: Year-round

SITES: 48

EACH SITE: Picnic table, fire ring, food-storage locker

ASSIGNMENT: First come, first served; reservations recommended in summer

REGISTRATION: Summer, at ranger station or reserve at reservecalifornia.com or 800-444-7275; fall–spring, self-register

FACILITIES: Heavily chlorinated tap water, pit toilets, wheelchair-accessible sites

PARKING: At site

FEE: $25 plus $8 nonrefundable reservation fee

ELEVATION: Near sea level

RESTRICTIONS:

PETS: On leash in campground only (not allowed on trails)

FIRES: In fire pits

ALCOHOL: No restrictions

VEHICLES: 3 vehicles per site; RVs up to 25 feet

OTHER: 10-day stay limit (20 per calendar year); do not feed wildlife; mountain lion, tick, and scorpion habitat

Some thought the wrong variety of eucalyptus was imported from Australia, but not so. Botanists have determined that eucalyptus planted in California has no natural pests, so it grows so fast it spindles. In Australia, insects slow trees' growth so their trunks don't spindle.

Today, Montaña de Oro State Park begins at the Morro Rock and goes south along a huge sandspit some 85 feet high. This is a prime area for hiking, picnicking, sunbathing, and swimming. You can get lost in little, private, sandy hollows in the dunes. On one side, you can see the sea, and on the other, Morro Bay, the largest, least-disturbed saltwater marsh in California. Bring a big backpack crammed with a blanket, water, food, and sunscreen, because the sandspit is an all-day affair.

Farther south, the sandspit gives way to more dunes that fall off to cliffs, flat sheet rock, and small cove beaches below. Park on Pecho Valley Road above at turnouts and hike over the dune and down. Again, bring supplies, because once you get down there, you won't want to leave.

Finally, south of park headquarters is an ancient wave-cut terrace with sharp, upended cliffs of Monterey shale that fall abruptly to the sea. Here and there, you'll spot accessible coves offering more sunbathing and wading (at low tide only). Don't miss Corallina Cove, about a mile south of the visitor center at the old Spooner Ranch House. At low tide, you can spot the plants and animals that live in the tidal pools. Obtain a free pamphlet and tidal schedule at the visitor center before you go.

East, off the coast, the park takes in about 8,000 acres of prime hiking, including Valencia Peak at 1,347 feet. From here, you can see the whole sweep of coast from Vandenberg Air Force Base (64 miles) in the south to Piedras Blancas (80 miles) in the north. I think Montaña de Oro provides the best spring hiking in California. By summer, it is too hot.

The two-loop Islay Creek Campground is in the canyon just behind Spooner's Cove, where big sailing ships once unloaded supplies and took on hides and tallow (for candles). Here, the canyon is narrow and runs along Islay Creek, which Spooner dammed up to run a waterwheel for power. All traffic goes by the neck of the canyon. It gets busy, so the best camping is in the back loop. As a trade-off, you'll have a longer walk to the beach from the back. Weekends are busy in the summer, so reserve early.

Camping in the canyon is close, but the atmosphere is friendly. The ranger station is right by the headquarters, and the information center is staffed by friendly locals. Montaña de Oro Campground makes you feel warm and safe. In summer, count on seeing lots of children. This means bicycles, skateboards, in-line skates, and the trill of youthful voices. Montaña de Oro is a prime family tent-camping vacation spot. If you can't handle that, head for the walk-in environmental campsites scattered in the park.

The tap water is technically potable; however, it is so heavily chlorinated that it is useful for washing only, so bring drinking water. Also, bring one of those plastic-bag showers to hang in a tree and sluice off the sand and salt. It wouldn't be a bad idea to bring a bucket to set by the tent for dipping sandy feet, and a brush and dust pan to keep sand out of your tent.

Montaña De Oro State Park: Islay Creek Campground

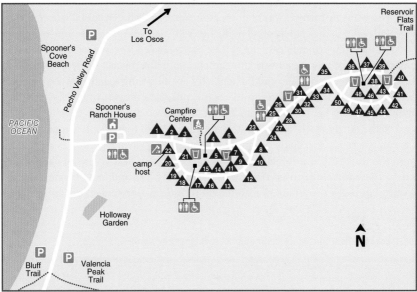

GETTING THERE

From Los Angeles, drive north about 174 miles on US 101 to the outskirts of San Luis Obispo. Turn left on Los Osos Valley Road and drive 11.5 west to Los Osos, where the road becomes Pecho Valley Road. Continue south 5 miles to Montaña de Oro State Park.

GPS COORDINATES: N35° 16' 26" W120° 52' 49"

9

Pinnacles Campground

Beauty ★★★★ / Privacy ★★★ / Spaciousness ★★★ / Quiet ★★★ / Security ★★★★★ / Cleanliness ★★★★★

Enjoy easy, hike-in access to Pinnacles National Park from this privately run campground.

Pinnacles National Park is a fascinating park. Miles of challenging trails thread over rock outcrops, along creeks, and even through caves. Unfortunately, the park's prime walk-in campground, on the west side of the park, was washed away in 1998's El Niño flooding, and there are no plans to rebuild. Fortunately, a wonderful, privately run campground sits inside the park's eastern boundary.

Pinnacles National Park has limited parking inside the park; by setting up a base camp at the campground, you can walk into the park or take a convenient shuttle bus. This translates to extra snuggle time in your sleeping bag, because even when the national monument's lots fill early, you won't be turned away on foot. From April to October, cool down after a grueling hike with a dip in the campground pool, then return to your campsite and lounge about.

Most of the campground's sites are at least partly shaded by coast live oaks, and there is a pleasant feeling of spaciousness at this campground. The owners really work on keeping the place clean, quiet, and safe, and the tent sites are all strung together at a good distance from the RV and group sites. On summer weekends, park rangers often host programs at the amphitheater. When we last camped here, we stayed at our campsite by the fire and listened to the ranger teach the kids in the audience how to howl like a coyote.

Camping here is particularly delightful in early spring, when wildflowers are breathtaking, and the trails at the national park are still cool. If you have the stamina for summer hiking on these mostly exposed trails, be sure to bring lots and lots of water, and get an early start. Pinnacles' most famous features are rock formations and caves, and you can get

Volcanic rock near Bear Gulch provides many rock-climbing opportunities.

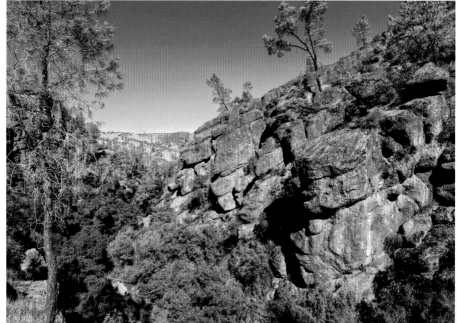

photographed by Steven P. Jordan/stevejordan.smugmug.com

KEY INFORMATION

LOCATION: 2400 CA 146, Paicines, CA 95043

CONTACT: 831-389-4485, nps.gov/pinn

OPERATED BY: Royal Elk Park Management

OPEN: Year-round

SITES: 134

EACH SITE: Picnic table, fire ring

ASSIGNMENT: Site-specific reservations accepted

REGISTRATION: At store (campground entrance) or reserve at recreation.gov or 877-444-6777

FACILITIES: Flush toilets, drinking water, firewood for sale, swimming pool (seasonal), coin-operated hot showers, store

PARKING: At site

FEE: $23 plus $9 nonrefundable reservation fee

ELEVATION: About 1,000'

RESTRICTIONS:

PETS: On leash in campground only (not allowed on trails)

FIRES: In established pits/rings/grills only; wood fires restricted during much of the year, but artificial logs are permitted; wood gathering prohibited

ALCOHOL: No restrictions

OTHER: Generators and amplified music are not permitted.

a short orientation to both on Bear Gulch Caves Trail, which departs from the Bear Gulch Nature Center, or a daylong tour de force on a hike combining Old Pinnacles and High Peaks Trails. The caves at Bear Gulch are closed for most of the year (to protect a threatened species of bat; call ahead for dates), while Balconies is generally open all year, unless high water floods the cave.

If you can manage it, the longer hike is highly recommended. Start at the campground with one flashlight or headlamp per person (believe me, you will stretch the bonds of a relationship attempting to share a flashlight), and walk west for 1.7 easy miles to a junction with the trail to Bear Gulch on the left and the trail to High Peaks on the right. Continue to the right for 0.6 mile, then arrive at the Chalone Creek trailhead. Pick your poison: High Peaks is steep and Balconies Caves is nearly level. I like to get to the cave early, so I prefer Balconies Caves, 2.3 miles from this trailhead. From Chalone Creek trailhead, hike west on Old Pinnacles Trail, following close to Chalone Creek, then reaching Balconies Cave. Here, the trail enters Balconies Cave—it's only 0.4 mile to daylight on the other side, but the cave is quite a thrill nonetheless, as you must follow the series of blazes and climb over some talus rocks through utter darkness.

After exiting the cave, blinking, it's another 0.6 mile to the Chaparral Ranger Station at the west side of the park. Be sure to fill up your water, then start to climb on Juniper Canyon Trail, a sharp ascent into the rock formations that give the park its name. From the High Peaks area, you'll likely see vultures and hawks, but also look for California condors, which have been reintroduced to the area. Return to Chalone Creek via the High Peaks Trail, then retrace your steps to the campground. Altogether, this hike is 11.5 miles, but the only really hard section is the part from Chaparral, the western trailhead, to Chalone Creek, and if you get an early enough start, you could shave off some miles by driving to the Chalone Creek trailhead.

Climbing is also permitted in the park—call ahead for current conditions and seasonal closures that protect nesting raptors. As you spend time in the park, be alert for wild pigs.

When my friend Kelly and I stopped at the far side of Balconies Cave for a restorative snack, we heard pigs grunting nearby and quickly left the area.

The campground store is small, so stock up in Hollister. In spring and summer you'll likely see fresh produce for sale at farm stands on the road from Gilroy to Hollister, but this rapidly expanding area south of San Jose has many large supermarkets and stores. Garlic is king around Gilroy (the garlic capital of the world), and if you believe that garlic does repel mosquitoes, as folk wisdom claims, you can stack the cards in your favor with a plethora of garlic-infused products available at stands and stores along US 101. Once you get to the campground you'll have to drive to the small settlements of Tres Piños and Paicines, about 18 miles north of the park, for a cooked meal at a restaurant. South of the campground and park, CA 25 is one of the most scenic drives in the area; this lonely road winds through grassland dotted with ranches, where there are far more cattle than people. I once saw a large herd of elk along the side of CA 25, and it barely made me blink—this part of San Benito County seems to linger with one foot in the past, when grizzly bears roamed the state.

Pinnacles Campground

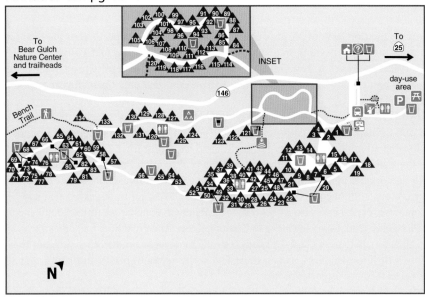

GETTING THERE

From US 101 in Gilroy, exit CA 25. Drive 13 miles south into Hollister, then follow CA 25 as it weaves through Hollister. Continue 31 miles south on CA 25, then turn right onto CA 146. Drive about 2 miles, then turn left into the campground.

GPS COORDINATES: N36° 29' 32" W121° 10' 42"

10

Point Mugu State Park:
SYCAMORE CANYON CAMPGROUND

Beauty ★★★★★ / Privacy ★★ / Spaciousness ★★★ / Quiet ★★★ / Security ★★★★★ / Cleanliness ★★★★★

Just outside Los Angeles, Point Mugu State Park is a jewel.

A school of dolphins pushing bait fish into the shore, working them around the rocky points, dolphin skin wet and black against the blue water—that was my first impression of Point Mugu State Park's Sycamore Canyon Campground. The beach is gorgeous, a white-sand jewel of a place to picnic, sun, and swim on an unspoiled stretch of coastline.

Later, I discovered that the Chumash tribe once lived in the canyon and believed that dolphins were their brothers. At one time, the Chumash lived on overpopulated islands to the west. Legend has it that their mother god told them to cross over the sea to the mainland by walking on a rainbow. The caveat was that they couldn't look down. Of course, some did and fell into the sea. But, the mother god took pity on them and turned them into dolphins.

The Chumash fished from canoes 25 feet long, lashed with sinew and caulked with asphalt from seeps. They gathered clams, oysters, and abalone along the shores and made soapstone bows inlaid with mother-of-pearl from the shells. They hunted and gathered food in the upper reaches of the canyon and lived a life of ease, culture, and bounty. Now we can camp where they lived before the Spanish came.

Like Malibu Creek State Park, Point Mugu State Park, and Sycamore Canyon Campground are heavily used, both for overnight camping and for day use. Buses of schoolkids come for the morning. Mountain bikers access the fire roads up in the canyon. And many

Take care as you walk along the rocky shore, as the smooth rocks may be slippery.

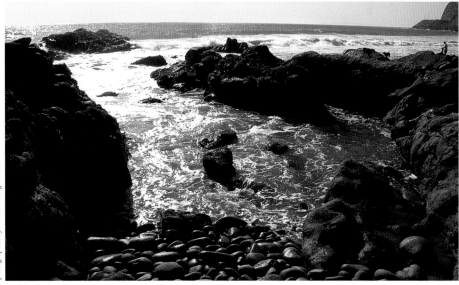

photographed by William Craig Tomlin

KEY INFORMATION

LOCATION: 9000 West Pacific Coast Highway, Malibu, CA 90265

CONTACT: 818-488-5223, parks.ca.gov

OPERATED BY: California State Parks

OPEN: Year-round

SITES: 56

EACH SITE: Picnic table, barbecue grill

ASSIGNMENT: First come, first served; reservations recommended in summer

REGISTRATION: At entrance or reserve at reservecalifornia.com or 800-444-7275

FACILITIES: Water, flush toilets, coin-operated showers

PARKING: At site

FEE: $45 plus $8 nonrefundable reservation fee

ELEVATION: Sea level

RESTRICTIONS:

PETS: On leash in campground only (not allowed on trails)

FIRES: Allowed (no wood gathering)

ALCOHOL: No restrictions

VEHICLES: RVs up to 31 feet

hikers come for the wildflowers. Still, the pristine beaches, rolling hills, savanna meadows, and the glorious canyon so close to the Greater Los Angeles Area make Sycamore Canyon a must-visit campground. Try to visit in the off-season, but watch the weather to schedule the best hiking days. Or, reserve ahead and hit the beach in the summer. The canyon is cool enough in summer for biking. Prime surf fishing is available off Thornhill Broome Beach, just up the road.

This is an excellent area for viewing monarch butterflies. They clump in the sycamores in the canyon and eat milkweed up in the meadows. Why don't seagulls descend on the

Starfish take up residence in the many tidepools beside the beach.

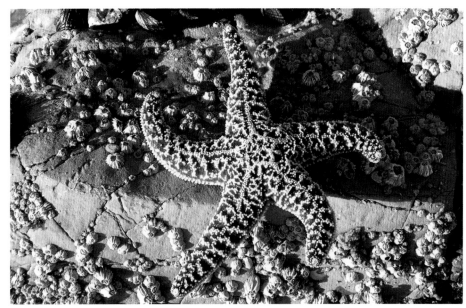

photographed by William Craig Tomlin

easily spotted, brightly decorated monarchs and have a big chow-down? Because milkweed is poisonous. Rasputin used it to knock off members of the Russian court. Milkweed is toxic enough that when birds pick up a milkweed-eating monarch, they feel sick and learn to leave them alone. The monarch's bright colors serve to alert the birds to eat at their own risk.

In Sycamore Canyon, you'll find many sycamores. You'll also find coast live oak and areas of chaparral and coastal shrub. Look for blue elderberry, wild rose, California bay laurel, purple sage, and of course, poison oak.

Like Malibu Creek State Park, there is a ranger headquarters at Point Mugu State Park, near Sycamore Campground. The park feels safe, well regulated, and well patrolled, which is comforting so close to a dense urban area. If you tire of Point Mugu's small beach, remember miles of beaches are just a short drive away. Neptune's Net, just south of the campground, is a good place to eat fish and chips or buy crab or lobster to grill. On some weekends, the outdoor patio restaurant can be overrun with biker gangs. Of course, upon close examination, the bikers look and act like very well-behaved middle-class Americans (and probably are!). They fit right in with the younger surfers and middle-aged campers.

You must plan a visit to Point Mugu and Sycamore Canyon. Watch the weather and avoid the June blahs. Beware of weather predictions calling for early-morning and late-afternoon fog along the coastline. And don't forget to make reservations. Don't expect the campground itself to be too scenic. Look to the sea, the sky, and the canyon for incredible vistas.

Point Mugu State Park: Sycamore Canyon Campground

GETTING THERE

From Los Angeles, drive 32 miles north up CA 1 or drive 16 miles south from Oxnard.

GPS COORDINATES: N34° 4' 23" W119° 0' 53"

11

Point Mugu State Park:
THORNHILL BROOME CAMPGROUND

Beauty ★★★★★ / Privacy ★★ / Spaciousness ★★★★★ / Quiet ★★ / Security ★★★ / Cleanliness ★★★★

Thornhill Broome is the only campground in SoCal that permits camping and campfires directly on the beach.

Thornhill Broome is the only campground in SoCal that permits camping right down to the waterline, which means you can set up your tent anywhere on the beach, unlike at McGrath or El Capitán, which only allow camping within sites above or behind the actual beach. The attraction of Thornhill Broome's genuine beach camping more than justifies the six-month waiting period needed to book one of the 68 sites during peak season.

From a geographic perspective, Thornhill Broome Beach lies between two points—Point Mugu to the northeast and a small point west of Sycamore Cove—and spans roughly 1.5 miles. The beach is rocky and the surf is usually very rough and exposed to open ocean swells, so on all but the flattest of days, swimming is advisable for experienced swimmers only. At the southeast end, opposite the ocean and across CA 1 (the Pacific Coast Highway), is a large sand dune. The northwest end terminates into Point Mugu, which features a large rocky formation. Just southeast of point Mugu and across CA 1 lies the entrance to La Jolla Canyon and the vast network of trails heading into the Santa Monica Mountains and Point Mugu State Park.

There's lots to do at Thornhill Broome Beach aside from typical beach activities such as sunbathing and swimming (with caution, of course). Hiking types will be pleased to know they're privy to many miles of trails accessible via La Jolla Canyon. Hard-core mountain

The sound of the ocean may help muffle the sound of cars on the highway behind you.

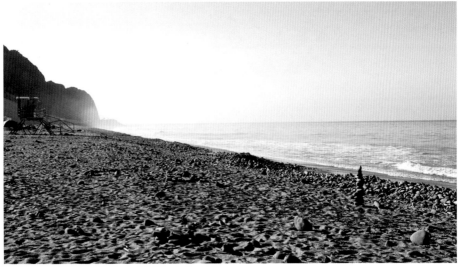

photographed by Steve White, Simi Valley, CA

KEY INFORMATION

LOCATION: 9000 West Pacific Coast Highway, Malibu, CA 90265

CONTACT: 310-457-8143, parks.ca.gov

OPERATED BY: California State Parks

OPEN: Year-round

SITES: 68

EACH SITE: Picnic table, fire ring

ASSIGNMENT: First come, first served or by reservation

REGISTRATION: Self-registration if park entrance station is closed or reserve at reservecalifornia.com or 800-444-7275

PARKING: No day use permitted; $4 parking fee for extra vehicles

FACILITIES: Toilets, running water, one cold- water shower

FEE: $35 plus $8 nonrefundable reservation fee

ELEVATION: Sea level

RESTRICTIONS:

PETS: On leash only and must remain inside tents or vehicles at night

FIRES: Permitted inside established fire rings

ALCOHOL: No restrictions

OTHER: Glass bottles are prohibited.

---

bikers have easy access to the trail networks of neighboring Big Sycamore Canyon. Surf fishermen can try their luck at the California halibut, California corbina, and barred surfperch teeming in the rough waters, and windsurfers will be pleased to find more than satisfactory conditions most of the year. Surfers and divers, on the other hand, will find little of interest at this locale and would be much happier at Leo Carrillo State Park (see page 25).

Though it's somewhat of a long shot, catching a keeper-sized halibut from shore at Thornhill Broome Beach can happen, but certain times of year are better than others. In the spring, the largest numbers of halibut enter shallow waters accessible to surf fishermen. Though these fish can be caught with bait, experienced anglers prefer casting artificial lures to cover the most area. A licensed fisherman cannot take halibut smaller than 22 inches in length. Taking undersized fish and/or fishing without a fishing license is an offense that carries serious penalties, so please play by the rules.

On really clear days, it's possible to see as many as four islands offshore on the horizon, but most days Anacapa Island, the smallest of the Channel Islands archipelago, will be visible to the west, behind which lies Santa Cruz Island. If the air is pristine, a small blip of land will be visible to the south. Easily confused with distant tanker ships, Santa Barbara Island is a lonely rock located more than 40 miles south of Thornhill Broome Beach. Seeing Catalina Island to the southeast is unlikely, but it is possible. Seeing the Channel Islands to the west is an enlightening experience for many—too many people in Los Angeles believe that Santa Catalina is the only island near shore in the vicinity of SoCal. In fact, there are eight islands in all, Santa Cruz being the largest.

As idyllic as Thornhill Broome Campground seems on paper, there are some downsides. The shoreline is more exposed to wind and high seas than most beaches in SoCal, meaning it can be pretty cold even when it's hot everywhere else. The waters aren't very inviting year-round, due to constant riptides and cold water, so amphibious campers may be unsatisfied. The trails at La Jolla Canyon and Big Sycamore are fantastic, but crossing the Pacific Coast Highway can be very dangerous, with no crosswalks available and cars roaring by at 60-plus miles per hour. The highway is also a source of constant noise, which can interfere with tranquility.

Campers needn't be choosy about site selection, because each of the 68 sites is smack-dab on the shoreline. If you intend to swim, pick a site between 1 and 10, as they are closest to the lone lifeguard tower. If you want easy access to La Jolla Canyon, a higher-numbered site is best, and the opposite is true for mountain bikers, because Big Sycamore Canyon is located around the point to the southeast.

All in all, Thornhill Broome may be the most genuine beach-camping experience north of Baja California. Sadly, you'll need considerable foresight to enjoy this place because of the six-month waiting period and the fact that rangers wait until very late to cancel reservations for no-shows. For sure, though, Thornhill Broome Beach is beautiful and worthy of any hassle.

Point Mugu State Park: Thornhill Broome Campground

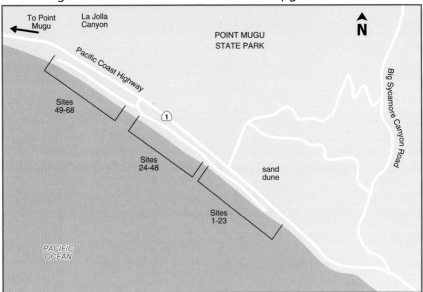

GETTING THERE

From Los Angeles, drive east on I-10 until it ends and becomes CA 1, or the Pacific Coast Highway. Driving west, stay on CA 1 for 32.7 miles until you reach Big Sycamore Canyon on the right, beyond Malibu. Thornhill Broome Beach is just around the corner, starting roughly 0.25 mile west of Sycamore Cove.

GPS COORDINATES: N34° 04' 55" W119° 01' 59"

12

Reyes Creek Campground

Beauty ★★★★ / Privacy ★★★ / Spaciousness ★★★ / Quiet ★★★ / Security ★★ / Cleanliness ★★★

This campground is dominated by Reyes Creek—every site is either creekside or near the creek.

Is there any sleep aid more potent than a rushing stream? The sound of rushing water always puts me to sleep quickly and keeps me there throughout the night, and that's exactly what happened at Reyes Creek. Even though we were camped a good distance from the water, the murmur of the creek provided the perfect volume of white noise for peaceful sleeping.

This campground is open all year and features generously spaced sites on and near the creek, where you can fish for rainbow trout or splash about in hot weather. Set in a wide, shallow bowl, the campground is dominated by scrub oak, manzanita, pinyon pine, chamise, silk-tassel bush, and near the creek, live oak, cottonwood, and alder. Small boulders and sandstone formations are prominent in the surrounding low, chaparral-studded hills. At just less than 4,000 feet, Reyes Creek Campground is best suited to spring and autumn camping, although there is a substantial amount of tree cover to shade you during the dusty months of summer, when a dip in the creek is just about mandatory. When we camped here in late April, the sites along the creek were full, but we were the only campers in the campground's largest loop, where a grassy, open meadow in the middle of the sites

Cedars and live oaks shade the campground's hiking trails.

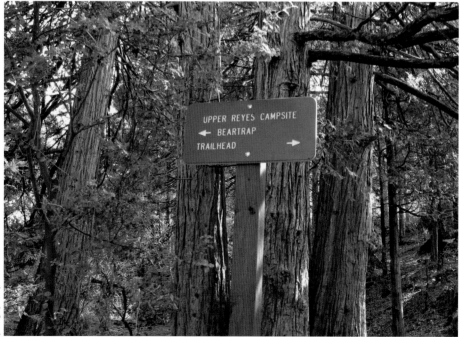

photographed by Pete Davis

KEY INFORMATION

LOCATION: 26901 Camp Scheideck Road, Maricopa, CA 93252

CONTACT: 805-968-6640, www.fs.usda.gov/lpnf

OPERATED BY: Los Padres National Forest

OPEN: Year-round

SITES: 30

EACH SITE: Picnic table, fire ring

ASSIGNMENT: First come, first served; no reservations

REGISTRATION: On site

FACILITIES: Pit toilets

PARKING: At site, additional vehicles $10/day

FEE: $20

ELEVATION: 3,960'

RESTRICTIONS:

PETS: On leash only

FIRES: In established pits/rings only; may be prohibited during high fire danger

ALCOHOL: No restrictions

---

is perfect for soaking up some sun in the afternoon. During the day the temperature was perfect, but it got seriously chilly once the sun dropped, and we ate breakfast while trying to keep our hands tucked in our jacket pockets. During the afternoon, a breeze rustled through the campground's pinyon pines, cottontail rabbits munched in the underbrush, and hummingbirds zipped around searching for nectar.

This is an old campground that feels slightly shabby (in a national forest kind of way); some of the picnic tables look like they were installed during the Kennedy administration. Just a few pieces of garbage strewn about a campsite can really make the area feel more rundown than it actually is, and I always volunteer a little light housekeeping before we pack up and leave any campsite. It usually takes only minutes to pick up any bottle caps and stray pieces of garbage, and I think that when campers arrive at a clean site, most are more likely to leave the site clean.

If you aren't content to fish or relax in your campsite, you can hike right from the campground. A short, paved, dead-end spur departs from the campground to the trailhead for Gene Marshall–Piedra Blanca Reyes Creek Trail, a narrow footpath running 18 miles southeast through the Sespe Wilderness, passing a string of backcountry campsites before ending at Middle Lion Campground. A few hours of out-and-back hiking on this trail earns an afternoon nap for sure.

Reyes Creek Campground is adjacent to a funky and rustic private camp, which sells ice and even cocktails, but for more substantial supplies, shop in Ojai—there are no other settlements in this area.

"Semiprimitive" campgrounds are plentiful in this part of Los Padres National Forest, where campground elevations range from around 2,000 feet (Wheeler Gorge) to 7,800 feet (Mount Pinos). There are numerous other camping options within a 20-mile radius of Reyes Creek Campground, most of which are small, nonreservable campgrounds with pit toilets, picnic tables, and fire rings, but no water. The campgrounds at the higher elevations, including Reyes Peak and Mount Pinos Campgrounds, are closed in winter, but two of Reyes Creek's nearest neighbors, Ozena and Pine Springs Campgrounds, are open year-round. On the way from Ojai, check out Rose Valley Campground on Sespe River Road, nine sites only 0.6 mile from Rose Valley Falls, or Reyes Peak Campground, six sites at 6,800 feet, a cooler summer choice. With the Los Padres National Forest map in hand, you could scout all of these campgrounds, settling on your favorite; if you live in Santa Barbara or the Greater Los Angeles Area, Reyes Creek and the other nearby campgrounds may quickly become your regular destination to escape the summer heat. Be sure to use extra caution with your campfires here, particularly in summer and autumn, when the surrounding forest is dry and prone to wildfires. Although open all year, Lockwood Valley Road and the road to the campground cross washes and may be impassable during wet weather—call ahead to check, and don't forget to bring your own water.

Reyes Creek Campground

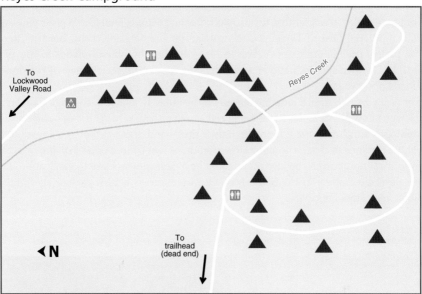

GETTING THERE

From Ojai, drive north on CA 33 for 36 miles, turn right onto Lockwood Valley Road, drive 3.2 miles, then turn right onto FS 7N11, signed to Reyes Creek Campground. Continue another 1.5 miles, past Scheideck Camp and Lodge, to the campground.

GPS COORDINATES: N34° 40' 45" W119° 18' 31"

13

⛺ Topanga State Park: MUSCH TRAIL CAMP

Beauty ★★★★ / Privacy ★★ / Spaciousness ★ / Quiet ★★★★ / Security ★★ / Cleanliness ★★★★

Just minutes from Los Angeles, go camping in the bohemian backwoods of Topanga Canyon.

Centered in the foothills of the bohemian hipster enclave known as Topanga Canyon, Musch Trail Camp is one of the Santa Monica Mountains' best-kept secrets. Of all the campsites detailed in this book, Musch Trail Camp is the closest, as the crow flies, to the big city of Los Angeles. Don't let that turn you off, though; Musch Trail Camp gives you a wonderfully unfiltered dose of Topanga Canyon's natural wonders and scenic beauty. There's a reason people pay big bucks on Airbnb to rent yurts and humble dwellings to stay in this place. It has its own special brand of magic that anyone can appreciate, even if you don't eat raw foods or do yoga.

For years, Musch Trail Camp has stayed off the radar. In fact, few Topanga Canyon residents even know about it, despite it being right in their backyard. This can be attributed to the campground's small size—there are only 8 sites—and, the fact that you'll need to hike in a short distance to reach the sites. However, these two factors don't explain everything. Perhaps it's simply hard to believe there could be a campsite so close to civilization. In the public psyche, camping in the Santa Monica Mountains is almost exclusively limited to Malibu Creek State Park.

A must-see view of the Pacific Ocean from Eagle Rock, the crown jewel of Topanga State Park

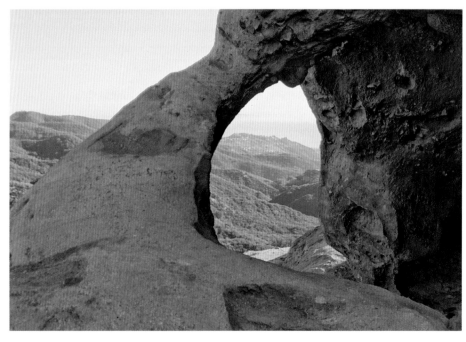

photographed by Charles Patterson

KEY INFORMATION

LOCATION: Trails leading to Musch Trail Camp can be found at Trippet Ranch: 20828 Entrada Road, Topanga, CA 90290

CONTACT: 310-455-2465, parks.ca.gov

OPERATED BY: National Park Service

OPEN: Year-round

SITES: 8

EACH SITE: Picnic table, fire ring

ASSIGNMENT: First come, first served

REGISTRATION: Self-registration if park entrance station is closed

PARKING: $10 per vehicle per day at Trippet Ranch

FACILITIES: Toilets, running water

FEE: $7

ELEVATION: 1,310'

RESTRICTIONS:
PETS: Prohibited

FIRES: Strictly prohibited

ALCOHOL: No restrictions

Once your skepticism goes away and you start to believe this campground is a real place, pack your stuff and go camping accordingly. Once you park your vehicle at Trippet Ranch (see directions on page 48). It's just a short walk from the parking lot via the Musch Trail. Once you've arrived at Musch Trail Camp you'll find picnic tables, bathrooms, and running water. It's one of the smallest officially sanctioned campgrounds in California, but also one of the sweetest.

Miles and miles of great trails to hike, some of Topanga's best, are easily accessed from Musch Trail Camp. Eagle Rock shouldn't be missed. You can get there by taking the Musch Trail northward from the camping area. After a few switchbacks, this singletrack terminates at East Topanga Fire Road, where you'll turn left and reach Eagle Rock after a short, moderate ascent. Fortunately, all of the major trails in this area are visible on Google Maps, so navigation is simple. Or you can simply hang out and take it all in. Musch Trail Camp is situated above much of Topanga's residential properties, so from the right vantage point, you might not see any sign of civilization as you stare out above the oak trees.

You can camp here year-round, but spring and early summer are probably best. In April and May, you'll be greeted with mild temperatures and full-bloom flora everywhere you look. In late summer, the warm-dry Santa Ana winds start to blow, making for night temps in the low 80s. Winter has its own delights, but temperatures can drop below freezing at night, so be prepared with appropriate clothing and sleeping arrangements.

The area has a few natural hazards to be aware of. Poison oak is common in shaded areas all over the Santa Monica Mountains. Get acquainted with the appearance of this nefarious vegetation, and avoid touching it at all costs. This plant is particularly dangerous when it loses its leaves in the fall and winter. In these seasons, avoid anything that looks like a brown twig sticking out of the ground. You should also be on the lookout for western diamondback rattlesnakes, particularly in summer and fall. These docile, beautiful, yet highly poisonous creatures aren't aggressive when unprovoked, but they can deliver a very nasty defensive bite if accidentally trampled on. If the unthinkable happens, seek medical attention immediately. There's also a very small population of mountain lions dispersed over the Santa Monica Mountains, but they're almost not worth mentioning. These big cats are so elusive they almost don't exist. Unless you're a deer or rabbit, you have nothing to worry about.

Groceries can be had at either of Topanga's markets—Topanga Creek General Store (141 S. Topanga Canyon Blvd., Topanga, CA 90290) or Fernwood Market (446 S. Topanga Canyon Blvd., Topanga, CA 90290). For anything else you might need, whether it be hippie jewelry, vintage clothing, incense, yoga lessons, fine art, or fancy dinners, look no further than the Topanga town center, roughly located at 122 N. Topanga Canyon Blvd., Topanga, CA 90290. Those apt to enjoy such attractions could easily get lost here, forgetting all notions of camping.

Topanga Canyon is a magical place, with a trippy, unique vibe that sets it apart from nearby, comparably stuffier, snobbier neighborhoods like Malibu, Pacific Palisades, Beverly Hills, and Brentwood. At Musch Trail Camp, you can experience all of Topanga's charms for pennies on the dollar. Do yourself a favor and visit this place. It's well worth it.

Topanga State Park: Musch Trail Camp

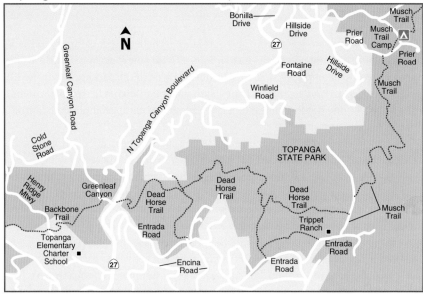

GETTING THERE

From Los Angeles, drive east on I-10 until it ends and becomes CA 1 (Pacific Coast Highway). Driving west, stay on CA 1 for 5.8 miles until you reach CA 27 (Topanga Canyon Blvd.) and turn right. Drive into Topanga Canyon for 4.7 miles, then turn right on Entrada Road. After 0.7 mile continue hard left on Entrada Road at the three-way intersection. The entrance to Trippet Ranch will be on your left, 0.4 mile from the intersection. The address is 20828 Entrada Road, Topanga, CA 90290.

GPS COORDINATES: N34° 06' 11" W118° 35' 02"

THE DESERT

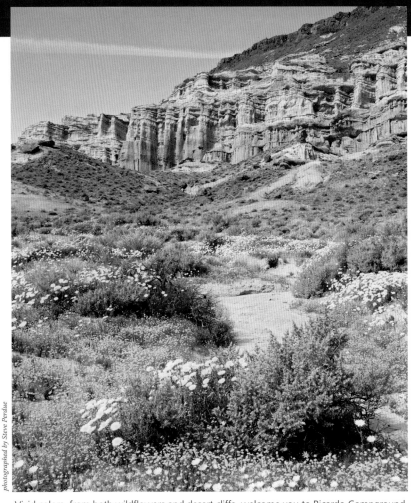

photographed by Steve Perdue

Vivid colors, from both wildflowers and desert cliffs, welcome you to Ricardo Campground (see page 62).

14

Anza-Borrego Desert State Park:
ARROYO SALADO PRIMITIVE CAMPGROUND

Beauty ★★★★★ / Privacy ★★★★★ / Spaciousness ★★★★★ / Quiet ★★★★★ / Security ★ / Cleanliness: ★★★★

Situated in malpais (badlands), Arroyo Salado features lizards, flowers, and the rainbow colors of the dunes.

Arroyo Salado is badlands camping. It is in malpais (badlands) in the huge Anza-Borrego Desert State Park (ABDSP), which has everything: palm-studded canyons, cactus gardens, mountain pinyon forests, hot springs, waterfalls, bighorn sheep, American Indian pictographs and petroglyphs, historic settler trails, stage stops, and ghost towns. A good way to come into Arroyo Salado is on CA 86, off I-10, via the cities of Indio and Coachella through the date palm orchards. Stop and have a date shake at one of the stands. Then, carry on along the shore past Salton City and turn east on County Road S22. Notice Travertine Point on the right and the wave terraces cut into the mountainsides—in 1905, the Salton basin was accidentally transformed into a huge lake by an overflow of one the Colorado River's canals. Near the wave terraces are traces of the American Indians who lived by the lake.

Now, you're in the malpais. This area is characterized by abrupt gullies with banks of sun-hardened clay, gravel-strewn sand, and strange shapes of clay. Red and yellow are the prevailing colors, with mud-hued grays and drabs for a background. After the winter rains, all the flowers bloom—flame-tipped ocotillo, verbena, desert sunflower, lavender, brittlebush, creosote bush, primrose, teddy-bear cholla, and beavertail cactus. The entrance to

The flat, desert land makes it easy to find a spot to pitch your tent.

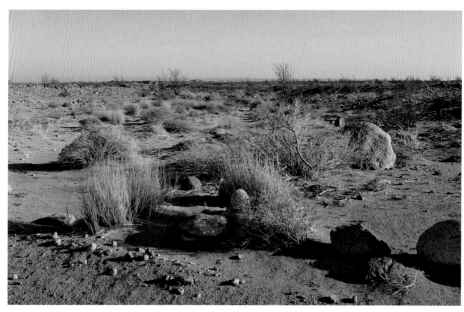

photographed by Four Herons Studios

KEY INFORMATION

LOCATION: CR S22, Borrego Springs, CA 92004

CONTACT: 760-767-5311, parks.ca.gov

OPERATED BY: California State Parks

OPEN: Year-round (avoid summer)

SITES: Open area

EACH SITE: No facilities

ASSIGNMENT: First come, first served; no reservations

REGISTRATION: Not required

FACILITIES: Vault toilet; bring plenty of water

PARKING: Some pullouts; otherwise, less than 10 feet off established dirt roads

FEE: None

ELEVATION: 880'

RESTRICTIONS:

PETS: On 6-foot maximum leash; not allowed on trails or in wilderness

FIRES: Only in existing fire rings, or in completely contained metal barbecues; must pack out ashes

ALCOHOL: No restrictions

VEHICLES: Suited for pickup campers

OTHER: Don't camp near water holes—wildlife depends on them for water; all vegetation (even deadwood) is protected.

the Arroyo Salado Primitive Campground is 11.8 miles on the left (or, from the opposite direction, 19 miles from the park headquarters in Borrego Springs). A metal sign reading ARROYO SALADO marks the campground. As with all signs in ABDSP, it is small and unannounced, so you have to be on your toes to see it. A turnaround past the entrance makes reapproaching a little easier.

An often-sandy road goes down the wash with various turnoffs where you can park your car and camp. Carry your tent up over the hummocks, and suddenly you'll be alone in untracked malpais. Anywhere is a good place to pitch a tent. The desert floor is clean and sandy. Sit down and listen to the wind, and look for lizards flitting over the rocks and dunes. Wait, and the desert comes to you.

The road continues down to Seventeen Palms Oasis, Una Palma, and Five Palms. None of these places has the number of palms their names advertise, but there is a spring at Seventeen Palms, as well as a visitor's register consisting of a wooden keg full of notes lodged in the palm fronds of two adjoining palm trees. Early travelers and prospectors began this desert post office. These considerate travelers also left a freshwater supply for those who followed. The saline water here is drinkable, although highly laxative. In the early 1900s, the famous British traveler J. Smeaton Chase came this way, noting of the water:

> Rice boiled in it was thoroughly disgusting in color and taste; no amount of sugar could render it more than just bearable. The tea had a dirty gray curdle and a flavor like bilge, and when I tried cocoa as an alternative the mixture promptly went black.

Past Seventeen Palms, the road continues south and connects with a network of roads in the Borrego Badlands. Don't go any farther unless you have a four-wheel-drive vehicle in good shape, and lots of water. You can camp anywhere you want in ABDSP as long as you don't park more than 10 feet off established dirt roads. Of course, you must carry out your garbage. However, a vault toilet spares campers the task of burying waste. No fires are allowed, unless you bring in wood and burn it in a fire ring or a metal container—a portable barbecue would be fine.

Remember, bring a lot of water; 1 gallon per day, per person should do it. It's not a bad idea to bring a collapsible shovel or sawed-off gardening shovel. If your vehicle gets stuck in the sand, it will be your best friend. Bring some old sheets and light rope. You can sit on one sheet and rig another for shade using the rope. Sleep under a sheet early in the night and get in your sleeping bag later when it gets cold.

To resupply or to escape the heat, go to Borrego Springs, where vendors sell grapefruit and oranges under shade trees on the traffic circle. Just up Palm Canyon Drive is the visitor center, where you can buy maps and books, and see exhibits. An easy 3-mile round-trip nature trail up Borrego Palm Canyon leaves from the Palm Canyon Campground 1 mile from the visitor center. Enjoy the park's more than 400,000 desert acres.

Arroyo Salado Primitive Campground

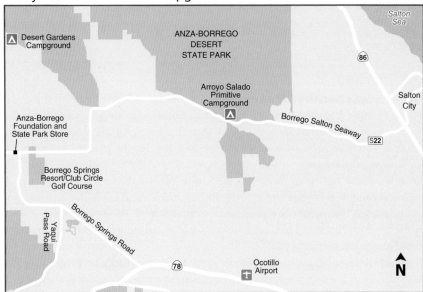

GETTING THERE

From Los Angeles, take I-10 east to CA 86. Head south to the junction with CR S22. Turn right and travel 11.8 miles to the entrance on the left. Or, take I-10 east to I-15 south to Temecula. Take CA 79 to the junction with CR S2. Take CR S2 to CR S22 to Borrego Springs. Drive 19 miles east of the visitor center on CR S22.

GPS COORDINATES: N 33°16' 51" W116° 05' 55"

15

Anza-Borrego Desert State Park:
BLAIR VALLEY PRIMITIVE CAMPGROUND

Beauty ★★★★★ / Privacy ★★★★★ / Spaciousness ★★★★★ / Quiet ★★★★★ / Security ★★ / Cleanliness ★★★★★

Here you'll find primitive tent camping in a valley full of wildflowers, American Indian pictographs, and mortars.

In the middle of March, I camped in Little Blair Valley on the edge of a tremendous meadow. The moon was so full that the tiny flowers sparkled from between the startlingly green grass. What a night!

I was alone until morning, when a couple drove by in a rental car. They were lost and looking for the American Indian pictographs. We consulted his map, then they were off in a cloud of dust. The rest of the morning it was just me, watching the sun move across the valley and rocks.

The County Road S2 turnoff to Little Blair Valley is 4 miles south of Scissors Crossing, about 31 miles from Anza-Borrego Desert State Park (ABDSP) headquarters in Borrego Springs. On the left, you'll see the tiny stake sign embossed with LITTLE BLAIR. The road, usually passable by all passenger cars, goes a mile or so over a ridge into the valley. Here, you'll encounter another stake sign indicating the CR S2 highway from which you just came. To the left is a wonderful area for camping in the soft meadow grass.

Clouds form large shadows over the Blair Valley.

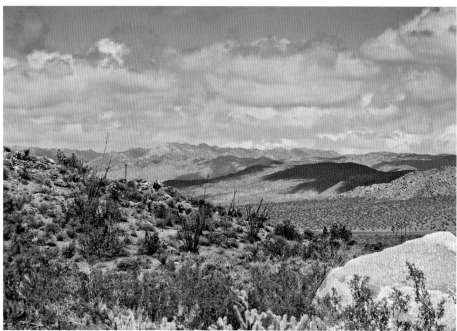

photographed by Shirley Savage, San Diego, CA

KEY INFORMATION

LOCATION: Little Blair Valley, Julian, CA 92036

CONTACT: 760-767-5311, parks.ca.gov

OPERATED BY: California State Parks

OPEN: Year-round (but avoid summer)

SITES: Open area

EACH SITE: No facilities

ASSIGNMENT: First come, first served; no reservations

REGISTRATION: Not required

FACILITIES: Vault toilets

PARKING: Some pullouts; otherwise, no more than 10 feet off established dirt roads

FEE: None

ELEVATION: 2,500'

RESTRICTIONS:

PETS: On 6-foot maximum leash; not allowed on trails or in wilderness

FIRES: Only in existing fire rings or in completely contained, metal barbecues; must pack out ashes

ALCOHOL: No restrictions

VEHICLES: Suited for pickup campers

OTHER: Don't camp near water holes— wildlife depends on them for water; all vegetation (even deadwood) is protected.

The road to the right of the CR S2 marker curls around the edge of the valley, passing several turnouts with many promising spots for parking and camping. Before you pick one, think about how the sun will travel and when you will want to be in the shade or sun.

From here, three short fun hikes are within easy range. Drive up to the head of Little Blair Valley and you'll see another stake signing the morteros. There is a parking area and a short 0.75-mile trail leading to large rocks filled with American Indian grinding holes. In these morteros (mortars), women pulverized coarse seeds and pods, such as mesquite beans, and made a pulp to be dried in the sun and used later for bread. Also, fine seeds and delicate plant parts were rubbed or lightly ground on smooth, polished patches of rock, known as slicks. The trail continues another mile or so east through a ruggedly beautiful canyon.

From the Morteros Trail parking lot, you can also follow a sign 0.1 mile to the Pictograph Trail. Usually passable, the 1.5-mile dirt road leads to the Pictograph Trail parking lot. From there, climb a ridge and go down the other side to a huge boulder painted in geometric red-and-yellow designs. Notice the distinct vegetation: juniper, white sage, and pinyon pine.

Go past the pictographs and see more American Indian morteros at the base of the ridge to the right. Continue down the wash and into Smuggler Canyon. When the canyon makes a sharp turn to the right, you'll see the Vallecito Valley and the Vallecito Stage Station from the edge of a steep drop.

Smuggler Canyon got its name from the laborers who came by boat from China, via the Sea of Cortez, to Mexicali. They were then smuggled up to the canyon to avoid law enforcement and angry locals. Once past the frontier, they worked in mines and on farms and railroads. A strenuous hike down Smuggler Canyon will lead you to CR S2, a few hundred yards east of Vallecito Stage Station. Arrange a pickup there, since the return is heavy going.

Drive 2 miles past the Morteros Trail parking lot into Blair Valley (not Little Blair Valley), and you'll see a signed turn to the left going to the Marshal South Home on Ghost

Mountain. Park in the lot just down the road and hike 1 mile straight up the mountain to see the ruins of the house.

In 1932, Marshal South and his wife, Tanya, built a house on top of the beautiful Ghost Mountain, which they called Yaquitepec. They saved rainwater in cisterns and ate yucca and agave like the local American Indians. Supplies were brought in by Model T from the town of Julian and carried up the mountain by mule or man. Marshal and Tanya raised three children and supported themselves by writing for *Desert* magazine. Finally, in a phrase that sends a chill down the spine of every married man, Tanya "tired of the eccentricities of her husband" and moved to San Diego, where she remarried.

From the parking lot, you can drive back to CR S2 through Blair Valley, passing several pullouts and some good camping sites. Blair Valley is regularly trafficked by RVs and tent campers. However, it is a good idea to check with the ABDSP headquarters about the conditions of the roads, especially after a rain.

Blair Valley Primitive Campground

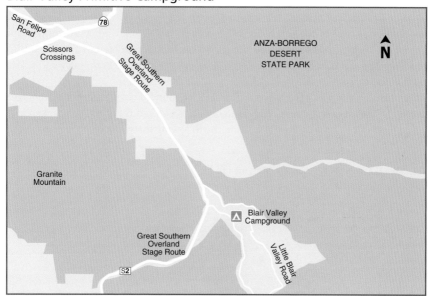

GETTING THERE

From Los Angeles, take I-10 east to I-15. Go south to Temecula. Take CA 79 east past Warner Springs to Julian. From Julian on CA 79, drive 12 miles east to CR S2. Go right 4 miles on CR S2 and find the stake marker LITTLE BLAIR on the left. Follow the dirt road about a mile to Little Blair Valley.

GPS COORDINATES: N33° 2' 7" W116° 24' 10"

16

Joshua Tree National Park:
WHITE TANK CAMPGROUND

Beauty ★★★★★ / Privacy ★★★ / Spaciousness ★★★ / Quiet ★★★★ / Security ★★★★ / Cleanliness ★★★★

White Tank has incredibly beautiful winter and spring camping, but don't get caught here in the summer.

Why is the arborescent tree yucca (*Yucca brevifolia*) called the Joshua tree? I have it on good authority that a group of Mormons was laboring across the trackless wastes, under a blazing sun, when they entered a *Yucca brevifolia* forest. Out of nowhere a cloud blocked the sun. In their ecstasy, the pioneers proclaimed the strange plants Joshua trees, referencing the Old Testament prophet who called on God to block the sun. Indeed, the tufted branches resemble an old, robed prophet imploring the heavens with raised hands.

I visited Joshua Tree National Park with a group of friends. We taxed our bones trekking up the strenuous trail to the top of Ryan Mountain. When my wife, who stopped speaking to me on the rigorous ascent, saw the snows on Mount San Jacinto and the Little San Bernardinos and the Lost Horse Valley spread below, she relented graciously and acknowledged that the carrot was worth the climb.

Then came White Tank Campground, where we found a cozy campsite in an alcove in the rocks. The pitch was soft and sandy, and boulders blocked the wind. We packed a lunch basket and set out to find White Tank using the following instructions:

Large granite boulders shade your tent from the hot sun.

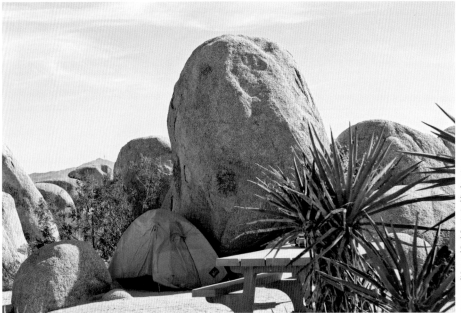

courtesy of National Park Service/public domain

KEY INFORMATION

LOCATION: 2 White Tank Campground Road, Twentynine Palms, CA 92277

CONTACT: 760-367-5500, nps.gov/jotr

OPERATED BY: National Park Service

OPEN: Year-round

SITES: 15

EACH SITE: Picnic table, fire ring

ASSIGNMENT: First come, first served; no reservations

REGISTRATION: At entrance

FACILITIES: Pit toilets, bring plenty of water

PARKING: At site

FEE: $15 plus $30 for a 7-day park entrance fee

ELEVATION: 3,800'

RESTRICTIONS:

PETS: On leash only

FIRES: In fire pits (bring your own firewood or charcoal)

ALCOHOL: No restrictions

VEHICLES: RVs up to 27 feet

OTHER: All vegetation in park protected; limit of 6 people, 2 tents, and 2 vehicles per site; no water provided

---

"Take the Arch Rock Trail. When you come to the sign that designates 'Arch,' stop and look around. To the south, 20 feet away, see the slabs of sandwiched rock. Climb over those, keeping the Arch Rock on the left, and you'll come down into sandy sheltered White Tank, a prime place for a picnic."

White Tank lived up to its billing. It was warm in the sun and cool under the huge rocks, and the sand was as white and clean as a Bahaman beach. What a lunch!

Afterward, we backtracked to the ARCH sign. Somewhere out there was Grand Tank, a body of water with colonies of fairy and tadpole shrimp. How did they get here? The friendly ranger at the park headquarters in Twentynine Palms told me their ancestors hitched a ride to Grand Tank on the feet of migrating ducks!

To find Grand Tank, head downhill from the ARCH sign and follow the trail that goes across a wash and up a hill. After a bit, the trail splits. We went left. "Follow the strong trail!" I urged my companions, who, when we reached a dead end, suggested I engrave that on my tombstone. Backing up, we climbed west to find the "strong trail" again. We saw birds diving into what we discovered were Grand Tank and the stream running south from it.

Vindicated at last, I identified white-winged doves and house finches circling the water. Grand Tank is about 15 feet deep. I looked in vain for the much vaunted, hitchhiking shrimp. As the day went on, I led my group of doubting Thomases south along the stream and safely back to camp.

That night there was a full moon. With field glasses we examined the figure on the lunar surface to see if it was indeed a long-eared rabbit as the Chinese believe or, in fact, the man widely publicized in my youth. Swayed perhaps because the next day was Easter, I conceded that it might be a rabbit after all.

A mile and a half back toward the park headquarters in Twentynine Palms is Belle Campground, just as charming as White Tank and as accessible to the California Riding and Hiking Trail. The trail, which crosses Cottonwood Springs Road between the two campgrounds, is best in early morning and evening, when twilight gives the flat desert rich hues and texture. Along with Ryan Campground in Lost Horse Valley, Belle and White Tank offer the best camping in Joshua Tree. Other campgrounds are overrun by RVs and rock climbers in fall and spring—the only times you want to be caught alive in this desert.

It's not a bad idea to check the weather report before you come to Joshua Tree. The Santa Ana winds come in the fall, and winds come from the coast in the winter, bringing rain. When it really blows, you must decide whether to tie your tent to the car or actually get inside the car. Sometimes it will blow for hours—sometimes days.

In any season, you can dine at the wonderfully idiosyncratic Twentynine Palms Inn adjacent to the park headquarters on the Oasis of Mara, Twentynine Palms' original raison d'être. Walk around and look at the ducks on the pond, the truck garden fenced by palm fronds, and guest cabins that once belonged to miners.

White Tank Campground

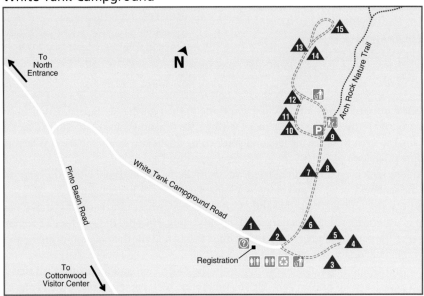

GETTING THERE

From Los Angeles, take I-10 east about 97 miles to Exit 117/CA 62. Go north and east on CA 62 for about 43 miles to Twentynine Palms. Turn right on the Utah Trail and travel 3.9 miles. Continue onto Park Boulevard and go 4.7 miles. Turn left on Pinto Basin Road and drive 2.7 miles. Turn left on White Tank Campground Road and you'll soon see the campground on your left.

GPS COORDINATES: N33° 29' 9" W116° 1' 0"

17

Mid Hills Campground

Beauty ★★★ / Privacy ★★★★★ / Spaciousness ★★★★ / Quiet ★★★★★ / Security ★★ / Cleanliness ★★★

Come to Mid Hills Campground for the spring bloom and back-road mountain biking.

The eastern half of the Mojave Desert isn't half as wild and woolly today as it was in 1826 when Jedediah Smith came through with a pack of angry Mojave on his trail. Ambushed crossing the Colorado River, Smith lost some of his trading party to Mojave war clubs before he forted up in a thicket of cottonwoods. With only five Kentucky rifles, Smith and his mountain men discouraged the Mojaves enough with pinpoint rifle fire to escape and run for their lives across the East Mojave Desert.

It was August 18 and hotter than Hades. Tormented by thirst, the men "found some relief from chewing slips of the Cabbage Pear," Smith wrote in his diary. Men dropped from exhaustion and could not go on until water could be found and brought back to them. "It seemed a more fitting abode for fiends than any living thing that belongs to our world," wrote James Ohio Pattie, another famous trapper of Smith's day. Traveling by night, the men spent the days beside springs that Smith vaguely remembered from his trip the year before. They followed the Old Mojave Trail—a trading route used by the Mojave for hundreds of years—and passed close by present-day Mid Hills Campground on their terrified flight across the desert wastes toward the Cajon Pass.

Nowadays, Mid Hills Campground is about the most pleasant place to spend some time in these parts. Set in rolling country among juniper and pinyon pine, Mid Hills is high

The unpaved access road and lack of utility hookups mean that you'll be sharing the campground only with fellow tent campers.

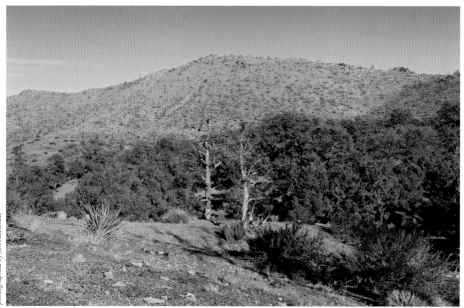

photographed by Jim McKenzie

KEY INFORMATION

LOCATION: Mojave National Preserve, Wild Horse Canyon Road, Essex, CA 92322

CONTACT: 760-928-2572, nps.gov/moja

OPERATED BY: National Park Service

OPEN: Year-round (forget summer, though)

SITES: 26

EACH SITE: Picnic table, fire ring

ASSIGNMENT: First come, first served; no reservations

REGISTRATION: At entrance

FACILITIES: Pit toilets, trash cans, water (usually)

PARKING: At site

FEE: $12

ELEVATION: 5,600'

RESTRICTIONS:

PETS: On leash only

FIRES: In fire rings

ALCOHOL: No restrictions

VEHICLES: 2 per site (the unpaved road to the campground is unsuitable for RVs)

OTHER: Bring firewood or charcoal.

enough to get snow, sometimes in May. I liked site 14 for its views of the mountains through the trees and the many places to pitch a tent. Also enticing are the sites situated on the edge of a drop, with a view of the vast Cima Dome and the Kelso Dunes to the south.

Between the Providence and New York Mountains, Mid Hills is the trailhead for the 8-mile hike to Hole-in-the-Wall Campground. Start at Mid Hills for a mostly downhill trek and arrange a return ride. A mile or so into the hike, there is a small, cold-water seep coming from beneath a dead juniper. I can imagine Jedediah Smith and his boys lying around there in the blazing sun waiting for the Mojave to beset them.

The trail features incredible views, and the land changes quickly from the pine–juniper forest to desert—with bright, delicate desert flowers for a short while in springtime. At the end of the hike, coming up a blind canyon, there are rings set in the rock that help get you over the steep sections of the hike.

Hole-in-the-Wall Campground is the only organized alternative to Mid Hills. When both campgrounds are full, campers may tent in "previously disturbed areas." This option gives you a couple thousand attractive campsites from which to choose. In fact, just around the corner from Hole-in-the-Wall Campground, you'll find a whole series of turnoffs on the incredibly scenic Wild Horse Canyon Road. Be sure to drive it—you'll see cholla and wildflowers growing on volcanic slopes and rocky mesa, sage, and the pinyon–juniper woodland of Mid Hills Campground.

When visiting the Mojave National Preserve, water is your paramount concern. Count on at least a gallon per person, per day. Phone the park before you leave to see which campground has water. When we visited, Hole-in-the-Wall had water, but Mid Hills didn't.

Gasoline is also scarce. Fill up when you can. It is illegal to burn anything you find in the preserve—even deadwood—so bring your own wood or charcoal. Wind is another consideration. Mid Hills is protected by trees and hills, but Hole-in-the-Wall is out in the open. Bring earplugs if you can't sleep through the noise of a tent flapping in the breeze.

Between Mitchell Caverns (tours available weekdays at 1:30 p.m., weekends at 10 a.m. and 3 p.m.); Kelso Dunes; Cinder Cone National Natural Landmark; Cima Dome; Fort Piute; Whiskey Pete's casino, hotel, restaurant, and truck stop just across the border in

Nevada; and the Mad Greek Cafe in Baker, you could easily spend a week around the Mojave National Preserve.

On the way to the Mojave National Preserve, stop at the California Welcome Center off I-15 (4 miles south of Barstow; 760-253-4782) for maps, guidebooks, and information. Spring is the season to visit Mojave National Preserve. Not only are the riots of flowers in bloom, but also the desert is scoured clean by winter, leaving a crust over the sand to keep down the dust.

Mid Hills Campground

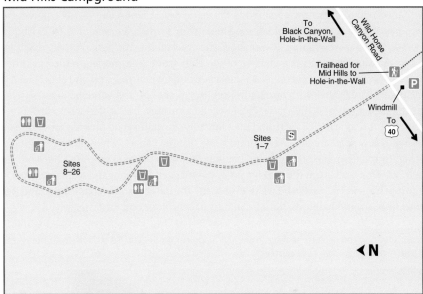

GETTING THERE

From Los Angeles, take I-10 east to I-15 north to I-40. Go east on I-40 for about 100 miles, then take the Essex Road exit and drive 10 miles north to Black Canyon Road. Take a slight right onto Black Canyon Road and drive 9 miles north. Turn left onto Wild Horse Road and follow the signs to the campground.

GPS COORDINATES: N35° 2' 37" W115° 23' 39"

18

Red Rock Canyon State Park:
RICARDO CAMPGROUND

Beauty ★★★★ / Privacy ★★ / Spaciousness ★★★ / Quiet ★★★ / Security ★★★ / Cleanliness ★★★★

Explore the Mojave Desert from Ricardo Campground, where Joshua trees stand sentry.

Once the location of gold rush prospecting and the backdrop for Hollywood movies, Red Rock Canyon State Park now preserves a dramatic desert landscape. Softly colored green, brown, peach, red, and white folded sandstone rock formations, sculpted by earthquakes and wind- and rain-weathering, tower above the desert floor. The park is bisected by a highway, and most people just get a glimpse of the cliffs from their moving vehicles. Although the desert seems drab and barren at 65 miles per hour, when you stop and slowly take it all in, the desert comes alive with fascinating geology, plant life, and animals.

In the desert, there is little privacy between campsites, but at Red Rock, Joshua trees, creosote shrubs, a variety of cacti, and the sandstone formations do provide some landscape buffering. Many sites are spaced a comfortable distance apart, while others are clustered more tightly together. If you don't mind hauling your stuff to your campsite, check out site 7, an easy 300-foot walk from the parking area. We snagged this spot and were rewarded with the most private desert campsite we've ever seen. The desert sand is coarse here, and it feels great to walk around barefoot, but be cautious of scorpions and rattlesnakes.

The park's historic and geologic features make this a popular destination, so arrive early to snag a spot in this first-come, first-serve campground.

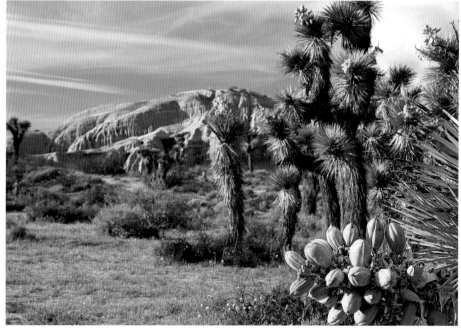

photographed by Steve Perdue

KEY INFORMATION

LOCATION: Abbott Dr., Cantil, CA 93519

CONTACT: 661-942-0662, parks.ca.gov

OPERATED BY: California State Parks

OPEN: Year-round, but too hot in summer

SITES: 50 sites for tents and RVs up to 30 feet

EACH SITE: Picnic table, fire ring

ASSIGNMENT: First come, first served; no reservations

REGISTRATION: At ranger station

FACILITIES: Pit toilets, drinking water, firewood for sale, 2 wheelchair-accessible sites

PARKING: At individual sites

FEE: $25

ELEVATION: 2,600'

RESTRICTIONS:

PETS: On leash in campground only (not allowed on trails)

FIRES: In established pits/rings only

ALCOHOL: No restrictions

The Mojave Desert is like an oven from late spring to autumn, and early spring is the favored season. When we visited in late April, there were still good displays of lingering wildflowers prominent on the bare, sandy desert floor near our campsite, including sand verbena, fiddle-necks, and golden gilia.

Serious stargazers camp here—park staff post sky charts on the campground information boards, and we saw folks with massive scopes, setting up at dusk. The campground's bowl-shaped orientation, tilted slightly uphill from the ranger station, allows good views of the sky, particularly to the north.

When you're exploring the desert, a good routine is to start your day early, hike when the temperatures are still cool, then return to camp for some serious afternoon lollygagging. Red Rock's easiest hikes are brief tours through the area, accompanied by interpretive guide pamphlets available at most trailheads. Introduce yourself to the area by exploring the visitor center exhibits at the ranger station, then walking the very short Ricardo Nature Trail, which begins across the parking lot from the ranger station. Stretch your legs more on Desert View Nature Trail, at the edge of the campground, or Hagen Canyon Trail, which starts from a trailhead right off the highway. To get to the other trailheads on the east side of the highway, you'll need to drive a short distance. Red Cliffs Trail requires only about 30 minutes to complete and is a good place to admire the park's namesake iron oxide–stained cliffs, as well as some of the area's best wildflowers in early spring. Another popular hike, indicated on the park map as Scenic Cliffs, is closed February–May to protect nesting birds; ask at the visitor center about this route's status.

In the afternoon, when the sun is high in the sky and the temperatures soar, you'll want to find some shade, so keep that in mind as you scope the campground for your site. On a hot afternoon we escaped to the shade of a small cluster of Joshua trees and tried to read, but were constantly distracted by birds. Wrens, finches, larks, flycatchers, and warblers are all frequently spotted in the park, along with two omnipresent desert birds: ravens and vultures. At night and early in the morning we heard an owl hooting nearby.

Once you exhaust the park's series of short hikes, there's not much else to do in the immediate area, so unless you're committed to total relaxation in a desert environment, you'll likely find a two- or three-night stay just right. If you want to go for a drive, head south and east of California City to the Desert Tortoise Natural Area, a Bureau of Land

Management–run preserve where you can look for tortoises on a 2-mile hike. Be sure to pick up all the food you need at Mojave. The Stater Bros. supermarket on CA 14 is the last chance for anything substantial, but you can pick up ice at the small store in Jawbone, a few miles south of the park. A BLM off-road vehicle area sprawls on the west of Red Rock Canyon, and from some sites you can occasionally hear the hum of dirt bikes. Some off-road enthusiasts set up base camp at Red Rock, but we found the jeep and dirt bike noise no more intrusive than that of the lumbering RVs and massive pickup trucks that are common to campgrounds these days.

Ricardo Campground

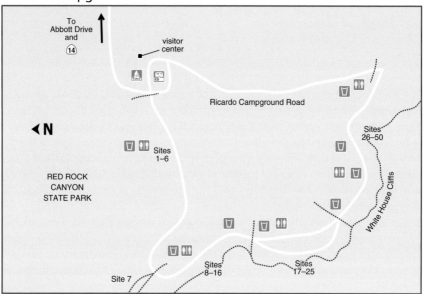

GETTING THERE

From the town of Mojave in Kern County, drive north on CA 14 for 24 miles. Turn left on Abbott Drive, following the sign for Ricardo Campground. Continue another 0.8 mile to the ranger station and campground.

GPS COORDINATES: N35° 22' 18" W117° 59' 34"

19

Saddleback Butte State Park Campground

Beauty ★★★ / Privacy ★★★ / Spaciousness ★★★ / Quiet ★★ / Security ★★★★★ / Cleanliness ★★★★

This is a fine first desert trip for children.

Saddleback Butte State Park is little known, well run, and very convenient to the Los Angeles area. It lies just over the hill on the Antelope Freeway, an oasis in the creeping suburbia of Antelope Valley. I like the park because of its proximity to Los Angeles. It's perfect for a quick desert-camping trip if you don't have time to drive to Joshua Tree National Park or Anza-Borrego Desert State Park.

The San Gabriel Mountains to the south block out the L.A. smog. You'll see wildflowers among the park's many Joshua trees February–May. In fact, the park was once called Joshua Tree State Park, but everyone confused it with Joshua Tree National Park, so they renamed it after Saddleback Butte, a mountain a few hundred yards to the east of the campground.

Look for horned larks and alligator lizards, as well as the golden eagle, desert tortoise, and the usual compendium of desert creatures. Examine the Joshua tree, which John C. Frémont dubbed the "most repulsive tree in the vegetable kingdom" in 1844. Later, J. Smeaton Chase likened the poor tree to "a misshapen pirate with belt, boots, hands, and teeth stuck full of daggers." Lighten up a bit, dudes. I think the Joshua tree is as beautiful as can be and as strong as it has to be to survive in a harsh environment.

When the sun sets, stargazing is a favorite pastime in the wide-open space of Antelope Valley.

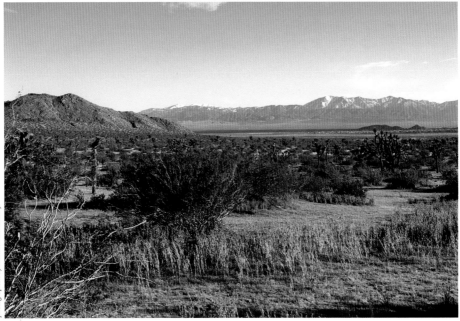

photographed by Michael K. McCarty

KEY INFORMATION

LOCATION: 17102 East Avenue J, Lancaster, CA 93535

CONTACT: 661-942-0662, parks.ca.gov

OPERATED BY: California State Parks

OPEN: Year-round

SITES: 50; 1 reserved for groups

EACH SITE: Barbecue grill, picnic table, fire ring, shade screen

ASSIGNMENT: First come, first served; no reservations for individual sites; group site is reservable

REGISTRATION: At site

FACILITIES: Water, flush toilets, dump station

PARKING: At site

FEE: $20

ELEVATION: 2,700'

RESTRICTIONS:

PETS: On leash in campground only

FIRES: In established rings only

ALCOHOL: No restrictions

VEHICLES: $5 for extra vehicle; RVs and trailers up to 30 feet; no hookups

The Joshua tree is a natural supermarket. Woodrats gnaw off the lower leaves to make nests. Weevils lay eggs in the tree's terminal bud, which causes the multiple branching effect. Yucca moths are the plants' sole pollinator, and in turn, lay their eggs in the flower. Butcher birds (loggerhead shrikes) hang their prey out to dry on the sharp leaves, and woodpeckers dig holes in the limbs looking for insects. In the past, American Indians ate the flowers, raw or roasted, and then ate the seedpods. They made sandals and carrying nets from the fiber in the leaves, and the roots were used to make dyes and medicines. In all, the Joshua tree is a useful plant. It's most attractive in spring, covered with and surrounded by flowers, or in winter, when the sunlight hits its tufted branches covered with snow.

The area around Saddleback Butte State Park was once antelope country. Imagine the Piute tribe on top of the 3,600-foot butte, scouting for herds of pronghorn antelope on the distant horizon. Then came the iron horse, the railroad, in the 1870s. Not only were there hordes of trigger-happy sportsmen on the train blazing away at anything that moved, but the pronghorn antelope also had their own fatal flaw: for some reason, they couldn't cross railroad tracks. Something in the pronghorn makeup wouldn't let them. So, unable to follow their normal grazing patterns, many starved to death.

The pronghorn are among the fastest animals in the world. Three feet high at the shoulder, the pronghorn can run 65 miles per hour in short bursts and 35 miles per hour for 4 miles. There are a few left in sagebrush country on the Modoc Plateau, but it's an uphill fight.

The trail up Saddleback Butte starts in the campground and moves due east up an easy grade, passing through creosote and Joshua trees. It winds around the alluvial fan and climbs up the saddle-shaped hunk of granite. From the top, you can see the other buttes in the area. All of them, including Saddleback Butte, are the tops of granite mountains silted up by the alluvial plain, which is Antelope Valley. To the north is Edwards Air Force Base, and farther west are Lancaster and the Antelope Valley California Poppy Reserve, where poppies blanket entire hillsides in brilliant orange. This area is worth a visit. Remember to phone ahead at 661-724-1180 to find out when the poppies are in bloom. From the Antelope Valley Freeway in Lancaster, take the Avenue I exit and drive 15 miles west to the reserve.

The Antelope Valley Indian Museum is also worth a stop. It is a folk museum of various American Indian tribes and houses a unique southwestern collection. It is open weekends from 11 a.m. to 4 p.m., mid-September to mid-June. To get to the museum, take 170th Street 3 miles south from the Park to Avenue M. Go west for 1 mile to the museum sign. You won't regret it.

Saddleback Butte State Park is first come, first served; however, the park is only really busy one or two weekends during peak flower time in the spring. Don't camp here in the summer. October and November are pleasant times to visit. Check the weather report and wind conditions before you leave; it can really blow here. In anticipation, there are windscreens by every campsite.

Saddleback Butte State Park Campground

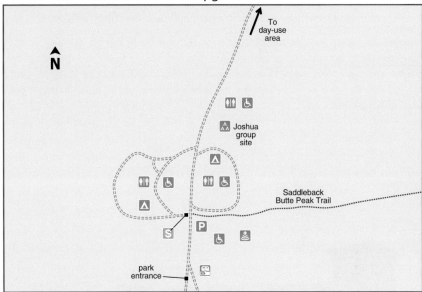

GETTING THERE

From Los Angeles, drive north on I-5 about 24 miles to Exit 162/CA 14. Take CA 14 north about 42 miles to Lancaster. Turn right (east) on Avenue J (County Highway N5) and drive 17 miles to the park entrance.

GPS COORDINATES: N34° 40' 36" W117° 49' 30"

20

Vallecito County Park Campground

Beauty ★★★ / Privacy ★★ / Spaciousness ★★★ / Quiet ★★★ / Security ★★★★★ / Cleanliness: ★★★★★

Vallecito County Park is good for children, winter camping, and Old West lore.

American Indians lived on the site of Vallecito County Park for thousands of years. Then came the Spanish conquistadors, Kit Carson and General Stephen Kearny, the forty-niners and the Conestoga wagons, and then, the stagecoaches. Vallecito oasis is on the main southern route west from St. Louis, which goes through Texas to avoid mountains and bad weather. The last water is near Yuma on the Colorado River, and then there's nothing but a hundred miles of trackless, dry wasteland.

One anonymous forty-niner quoted on a park billboard describes Vallecito this way:

Imagine the weary traveler, ragged and dirty, surrounded by barren, burning sands, with no green thing upon which to rest his eye. See him toiling to ascend the sandy rise. He reaches the top and in the distance he sees the green countenance of Vallecito. Gratitude to God fills his heart when he reaches the spot where he can lie down in green pastures and refresh himself.

The Vallecito Stage Station was built circa 1852 from sod cut from salt grass and restored in the early 1930s.

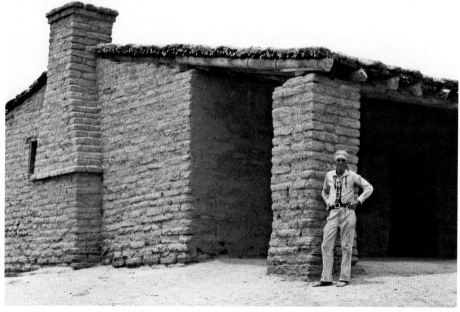

Marshal South Collection, courtesy of Diana Lindsay

KEY INFORMATION

LOCATION: 37349 Great South Stage Route 1849, Julian, CA 92036

OPERATED BY: San Diego County Department of Parks and Recreation

CONTACT: 760-765-1188, sdparks.org

OPEN: Labor Day weekend–Memorial Day weekend

SITES: 44, plus 8 equestrian sites with corrals

EACH SITE: Picnic table, barbecue stove, fire ring

ASSIGNMENT: First come, first served or by reservation

REGISTRATION: By entrance; for reservations call 858-565-3600 or visit reservations.sdparks.org

FACILITIES: Water, flush toilets, playground

PARKING: At individual sites

FEE: $22

ELEVATION: 1,500 feet

RESTRICTIONS:

PETS: On 6-foot leash; must be attended at all times; $1 fee

FIRES: In established barbecue stoves or fire rings

VEHICLES: RVs or trailers

ALCOHOL: Beer and wine; nothing over 40 proof

OTHER: No generators

Ripping through the desert in an air-conditioned car, you won't get quite the same sensation, but Vallecito is truly a magical spot. Surrounded by mountains of heat-blasted rock, Vallecito is soft, green, and filled with wildlife. Behind the campground is a privately owned preserve, a mesquite forest alive with bees and birds.

The campground is simple. Under the trees, near the restored stage station and cemetery on the only high ground, sit the 22 tent-only spots—well away from the RV and trailer area. The restrooms are simple and clean. The ranger is on top of everything. This is a beautiful, well-run camp. It is a perfect place to come with children for a first-time camping trip or to frame nights spent camping in Anza-Borrego Desert State Park primitive campsites.

A playground entertains little ones. You can spot rabbits hopping through the campground, as well as roadrunners, lizards, and quail. Bring binoculars and a bird book. For meals, bring charcoal and items to grill. If you forget, you can buy supplies at the two stores nearby—Butterfield Ranch and Agua Caliente. Both places also have swimming pools available for a small fee.

The reconstructed stage station is fascinating and full of history involving hauntings, lost gold, and murder. Reports say that a man rode his white horse into the station one night and shot his brother dead at the bar. Another story tells of a young woman who came off the stagecoach and expired in the station. An elaborate wedding dress was found in her baggage. She was buried in it, and sometimes her apparition is seen wafting through the rooms of the stage station at dusk. Some days, hundreds of Conestoga wagons camped around the station, as the oxen and settlers gathered strength for the final push over the mountains.

The stagecoaches ran 24 hours a day. At night a man on horseback rode ahead, carrying a lantern to light the way. A six-horse team pulled the stage. There were quick stops to change horses and only one meal per day for the passengers. The 2,800-mile trip from St. Louis to San Francisco took 24 days. Imagine more than 100 miles per day in a stagecoach with no springs!

Nearby hiking is available. You can bushwhack in the desert across the road or trek up the sandy wash of Smuggler Canyon. A short car ride away, you'll find Emigrant Trail and Blair Valley to the north, and trailheads at Bow Willow in the south. A good gem-hunting trip is located south, on CR S2 almost to Ocotillo. On the left is Shell Canyon Road. Drive as far as you can, then hike. The canyon is filled with fossil shells and onyx. Go east on CR S80 for 4 miles past Ocotillo and turn left on Painted Gorge Road. Again, be careful of the sand. There are agate and jasper immediately on the left and fossils in the hills to the right farther up the mountain. This is a good hike even if you aren't interested in gems.

Vallecito County Park Campground

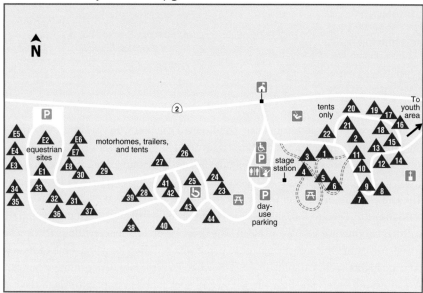

GETTING THERE

From San Diego take I-8 east about 35 miles. Take Exit 40 for CA 79 N toward Julian. Turn left onto CA 79 and drive 23 miles. Turn right onto CA 78 and travel a little over 11 miles through Banner to Scissors Crossing. Turn right onto CR S2 and drive 17.8 miles to the park.

GPS COORDINATES: N32° 58' 31" W116° 21' 1"

THE NORTHERN SIERRAS

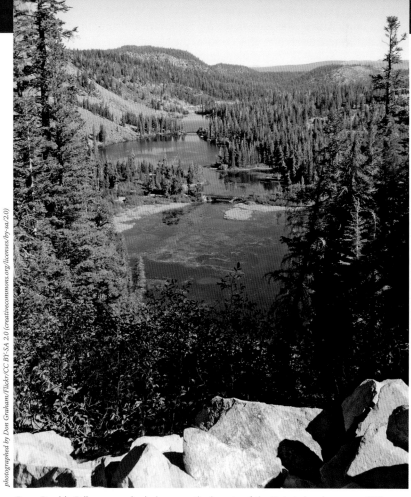

From Double Falls you can look down on the beauty of the Twin Lakes (see page 133).

21

Atwell Mill Campground

Beauty ★★★★★ / Privacy ★★★★★ / Spaciousness ★★★★★ / Quiet ★★★★ / Security ★★★★★ /
Cleanliness ★★★★★

This is one of the two best backcountry campgrounds in Sequoia National Park.

Drive through torrid Visalia on any July afternoon and you'll know why the Yokut and Monache tribes fought over the summer camps by Atwell Mills, where it is pleasant during the day and cool at night. They built little, round thatched houses and carpeted the floor with oak leaves and ferns. The women gathered most of the food, and the men spent most of their time in the sweathouse. Summer was a time of plenty for them, with pine nuts, fish, manzanita cider, wild tobacco, and an occasional deer. The deer were stalked by one man alone, wearing a deer disguise and using arrows poisoned with rattlesnake venom. The American Indians here led a great life, but it went like the wind when the white man appeared on the scene, hot after the riches located in the Mineral King Valley.

The road up to Atwell Mill follows the old American Indian trail. It's steep, but near Atwell Mill the ground levels out. This is one of the few areas around flat enough to camp and work on. A. J. Atwell of Visalia thought so, and built a small sawmill in the meadow

Remnants of the late 19th-century sawmill can be found near the campground; wood from Atwell Mill was used to build cabins for forty-niners.

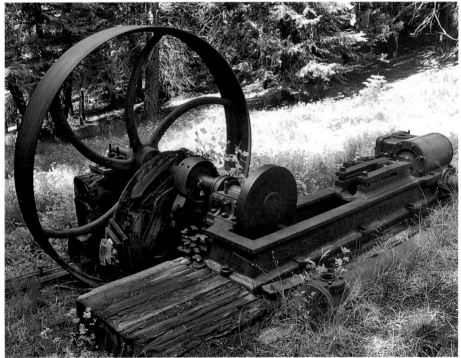

photographed by Clare and Ben

KEY INFORMATION

LOCATION: 19 miles east of CA 198 on Mineral King Road, Three Rivers, CA 93271

CONTACT: 559-565-3341, nps.gov/seki

OPERATED BY: National Park Service

OPEN: Memorial Day–October 31 (weather permitting)

SITES: 21

EACH SITE: Picnic table, fire ring, bear box

ASSIGNMENT: First come, first served; no reservations

REGISTRATION: At entrance

FACILITIES: Water, pit toilets, wheelchair-accessible sites

PARKING: At site

FEE: $12 plus $30 for a 7-day park entrance fee

ELEVATION: 6,650'

RESTRICTIONS:

PETS: On leash in campground only (not allowed on trails)

FIRES: Allowed in fire pits; may be prohibited when fire danger is high

ALCOHOL: No restrictions

VEHICLES: 1 vehicle per site; 6 people maximum per site; no RVs or trailers

OTHER: Don't leave food out, use bear boxes; 14-day stay limit

below the campground. You can still see the remains of the mill's steam engine near the stumps of the giant sequoias it helped reduce to shingles, grape stakes, and fence posts.

Steam engines tore their way through the American West. Anywhere there was fuel for the boiler, the engine could do the work of hundreds of men. Some American Indians thought engines were a breed of devil, and for them I think that was true.

Folks knew how to build a steam engine for a thousand years before they could make iron durable enough for steam boilers. Finally, in England in 1600, a blacksmith experimented with burning coke in order to make a better frying pan and discovered the process that produces high-grade iron. That discovery ultimately enabled deforestation at Atwell Mill.

Still, there's a magic to Atwell Mill. It's in the scarred stumps more than 100 years old. It's in the young sequoias reaching up in the shade of cedars, pines, and white firs. This is classic mountain camping.

All winter, the campsites are cleansed by 20 feet of snow. In the summer, the air smells clean and rich with the odor of redwood and pine. Walk up the little ridge above the campground and watch the sun set on the mountains across the Kaweah River. Or better yet, head down the Atwell-Hockett Trail between campsites 16 and 17. The trail passes the supine steam engine on the right and heads over the hill. About 100 yards from the metal sign banning firearms and dogs, go to the right, about 30 yards down, to the famous American Indian bathtubs. The rock outcropping there is a great place to have lunch or a sundowner. There, manzanita open up the forest to give you a great view of the mountains and sky.

Back on the main trail, carry on past little Deadwood Creek to East Fork of the Kaweah River gorge with its giant sequoias and mist kicked up by the falls. Rough trails head up either side of the gorge for more private picnicking and sunning spots. Or, keep walking the many miles up to Hockett Meadows.

Another good hike is up the Atwell Redwood Trail. From the campground, walk back down the Mineral King Road you drove up on and find the trailhead at a curve about 500 yards down. Hike up the mountain into the Atwell Grove sequoias. Three of these trees are gigantic. At their feet are the bracken fern that the American Indians used to carpet the floors of their houses. Keep hiking up and to the left along the ridge to Paradise Peak. The hike is about 9 miles round-trip and should take you all day.

Remember, when you leave Three Rivers you are bidding adieu to ice-and-beer country. So, ice up. Remember, block ice lasts about three days compared to cube ice's one day.

The sign where the Mineral King Road takes off from CA 198 should tell you if Atwell Mills and Cold Springs have campsites available. However, this sign is not always up to date, so phone the ranger station in Mineral King at 559-565-3341 to make sure. It is a 3-hour round-trip, so you don't want to arrive and not find a campsite. On the Mineral King Road turn your lights on. It helps traffic see you a split second earlier, which means a lot on this hairy road. Bring bug repellent in August to deter biting pests. And remember to use the bear boxes!

Atwell Mill Campground

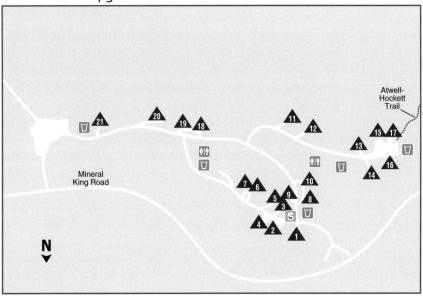

GETTING THERE

From Los Angeles, take I-5 north over the Tejon Pass to CA 99. Drive north on CA 99 past Bakersfield. Take CA 65 north to Exeter. Turn right (east) on CA 198 to Three Rivers. Three miles past Three Rivers turn right onto Mineral King Road. It's about 19 miles to Atwell Mill. Plan on the 19-mile trip taking about 1.5 hours.

GPS COORDINATES: N36° 27' 51" W118° 40' 05"

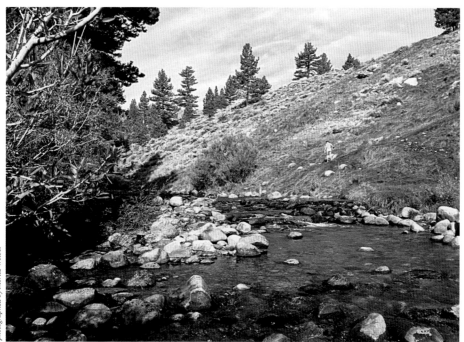

22

Buckeye Campground

Beauty ★★★★★ / Privacy ★★★★★ / Spaciousness ★★★★★ / Quiet ★★★★★ / Security ★★★★★ / Cleanliness ★★★★★

Come for fishing, hiking, the magnificent rocky slopes, and far-off glaciers.

All roads that lead to Buckeye Campground also pass the Burger Barn in Bridgeport. Anytime is a good time for an everything-on-it burger, wrapped in wax paper, at the outside tables of this ageless monument to roadside dining. Historic Bridgeport's Burger Barn is a famous relic of Americana. One assumes that the lean, tasty burger meat comes from close relatives of the sleek cattle grazing in the knee-deep grass around town. After all, this is cattle country. In Bridgeport, the heart of the Old West steadily beats.

The campground has four loops. The first loop you come to on the left houses sites 42–68. Continue up the hill to find the other three loops. Two have pit toilets, and the other has flush toilets but was closed the last time I was up there.

At 7,000 feet, Buckeye is idyllic Sierra Nevada camping. The air smells of pine, dust, and cold, rushing water. The mountain wildflowers grow from the sandy, needled floor among the sage. You look up and see the rocky slopes and, farther on, the white of the glaciers on the peaks: it's cowboy country. A horse trail cuts right by the camp. The sites are mostly unoccupied; the pitches are scoured clean by the winter. This is an excellent place to camp.

Buckeye Creek runs right past the campground.

photographed by Moritz Weibel

KEY INFORMATION

LOCATION: Humboldt-Toiyabe National Forest, Buckeye Road, Bridgeport, CA 93517

CONTACT: 760-932-7070, www.fs.usda.gov/htnf

OPERATED BY: U.S. Forest Service

OPEN: May–October (depending on road and weather conditions)

SITES: 68

EACH SITE: Picnic table, fire ring

ASSIGNMENT: First come, first served; no reservations

REGISTRATION: At entrance to each loop

FACILITIES: Flush and vault toilets, drinking water

PARKING: At individual site

FEE: $18

ELEVATION: 7,500'

RESTRICTIONS:

PETS: On leash only

FIRES: In fire ring

ALCOHOL: No restrictions

VEHICLES: RVs up to 30 feet

OTHER: Don't leave food out.

Fishing is not bad on Buckeye Creek between the two bridges—that's where the fish are stocked. You can hike on over to Twin Lakes and rent a boat. Go for the big brown trout. In 1987 somebody caught the state record, a 26.8 pounder, here. However, most of the folks I saw with fish had caught little rainbows. The water-skiing on Upper Twin scares away some of the trout, so the best fishing is on Lower Twin. I talked with one old-timer who said the best time to come for the browns is in May, when it is cold and windy. Troll with rapalas (three- to four-inch minnow-shaped lures), he advised. I threw in some salmon eggs and didn't get a nibble.

Another big draw at Buckeye Campground is the hot springs. They are by the stream down from the campground. It's best to get in your car and drive down the hill. Take your first left and climb a slight hill. There is a slanting parking area immediately on the right. Climb down the steep slope to the hot pools by the river below. This can be fun. Wear shoes with some traction since the footing is slippery. Sometimes the pools are empty, sometimes filled with fun-loving folks. Last time I was there, one pool was occupied by a lone, naked, whale-like chap who looked boiled-lobster pink. I chose to wear bathing apparel. I sat first in the hot pool, then sat in Buckeye Creek to cool off.

Good hiking can be had right out of camp. Buckeye Campground is in a V between the two branches of Buckeye Creek. The two hikes follow the two branches upstream and ultimately swing around and join one another, so you can make up to a 16-mile loop. Bring fishing gear since there are elusive brown trout and rainbow in the upper reaches; use local worms and try the pools behind beaver dams. The trailhead to the two hikes is up above the campground loops. Just walk up the access road (newly tarred and graveled) and it will dead-end into a horse corral and the trailhead (see the map posted there).

One trailheads west along the right-hand branch of Buckeye Creek. This trail follows an erstwhile wagon road through flowered meadows and pine forest. The trail up the left-hand branch of Buckeye Creek can be accessed from the campground's left-hand loops (looking west). Just walk to the creek and head up the fisherman's trail. Otherwise, walk from the trailhead a few hundred yards until the trail winds left up a ridge to the stream. The wildflowers in July were all over the place—lupine, shooting star, paintbrush. Watch the campground notice board for ranger wildflower nature walks—they are fun.

Bring ice—the nearest supplies are at Doc and Al's, or Bridgeport. Think about cooling your drinks in the stream. Or buy a cheap Styrofoam cooler, fill it with ice, duct-tape it shut, and put it in a cool place. Mind the bears. Put all of your food in the car trunk when you leave camp. Bears are busy tending their cubs and looking for chow during camping season. By fall, bears max out, eating 20,000 calories every day in preparation for hibernation.

Good side trips from Buckeye are to Bodie (bring food and water), Mono Lake, and the Virginia Creek Settlement (once part of Dogtown, a gold-rush mining camp) for a look around and a meal. Go gem hunting near Bridgeport. Head 3.3 miles north from Bridgeport on CA 182, and turn right on FS 46. Head out exploring (avoid any active mines) for quartz crystals, chalcopyrite, and pyrite.

Buckeye Campground

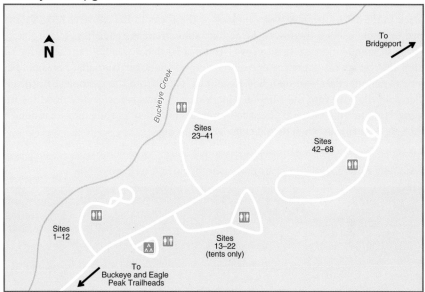

GETTING THERE

From Bridgeport, take Twin Lakes Road southwest a little over 7 miles to Buckeye Road. Turn right onto Buckeye Road by Doc and Al's Resort and travel about 4 miles on the dirt road to the campground.

GPS COORDINATES: N38° 14' 22" W119° 20' 53"

23

Cold Springs Campground

Beauty ★★★★★ / Privacy ★★★★★ / Spaciousness ★★★★★ / Quiet ★★★★★ / Security ★★★★★ /
Cleanliness ★★★★★

Cold Springs is the most beautiful campground in the adjacent Sequoia & Kings Canyon National Parks.

Cold Springs Campground is arguably the most beautiful campground in Southern California. Down by the gorgeous Kaweah River, this campground is situated in the shadows of Sawtooth and Mineral Peaks, Needham and Rainbow Mountains, and to the south, Miners Ridge. Winter scours out the valley so it feels brand new every summer. A waterfall cuts through the walk-in camping area. The rush of the water is white noise; you'll sleep like a baby. I love this campground.

Back in the 1870s, miners took one look at the rocks in the Mineral King Valley and rushed in. What excited them was the contact zone between reddish metamorphic rocks and grayish granite. So sure of silver was Thomas Fowler, a wealthy rancher from Tulare County, that he bet his entire fortune on his Empire Mine, boasting that he would pay off America's national debt and then buy Ireland to free it from the tyrannical British. First, Fowler built the road into the Mineral King Valley. A local reporter described the mine's opening: "I doubt that General Grant felt more proud when he rode into Richmond than did honest Tom Fowler when he rode into Mineral King."

Campers rest easy here, lullabied by the rushing water of the East Fork Kaweah River.

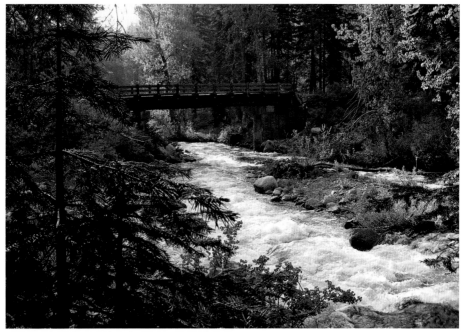

KEY INFORMATION

LOCATION: 23 miles east of CA 198 on Mineral King Road, Three Rivers, CA 93271

CONTACT: 559-565-3341, nps.gov/seki

OPERATED BY: National Park Service

OPEN: Memorial Day–late October (weather permitting)

SITES: 40

EACH SITE: Picnic table, fire ring, bear box

ASSIGNMENT: First come, first served; no reservations

REGISTRATION: At entrance

FACILITIES: Water, pit toilets, coin-operated showers, wheelchair-accessible sites

PARKING: At site

FEE: $12 plus $20 for a 7-day park entrance fee

ELEVATION: 7,500'

RESTRICTIONS:

PETS: On leash in campground only (not allowed on trails)

FIRES: Allowed in fire pits; fires may be restricted during high fire season

ALCOHOL: No restrictions

VEHICLES: No RVs or trailers

OTHER: No harming marmots; keep food in bear boxes, not in tents or cars; 14-day stay limit.

Of course, the mine went bust. Avalanches swept away the mine, the town that popped up around it, and the mile-long bucket tramway to the stamp mill in the valley. All that was left of Fowler's dream was the road, and folks used it to get away from the brutal heat in the Central Valley below. In 1893, the federal government declared the area part of the Sierra Forest Preserve.

In the 1960s, the U.S. Forest Service considered building a major ski resort in the Mineral King Valley. The Walt Disney Corporation proposed a resort with a skiing capacity of 10,000 persons daily. Widespread opposition and lawsuits from environmental groups ensued, and finally, in 1978, Congress made the Mineral King Valley part of Sequoia National Park.

Now Mineral King is famous for its marmots. These little devils have a penchant for gnawing on auto parts from early spring to about mid-July. They chew on hoses, fan belts, and electrical wiring. Some people bring chicken wire to put around their cars. Unless you park on a hard surface and seal the edges of the wire with piled rocks, so the marmots can't dig their way in, the chicken wire just makes a big marmot playpen. In springtime, leave your car in the hikers' parking lot in Atwell Mill Campground, and get a lift up to Mineral King. As the summer progresses, the chewing ends, and marmot-safe parking reaches higher altitudes until it is safe to park at the trailheads in Mineral King. It's a good idea to phone the rangers and ask about the latest on marmot activity. You don't want to pay $250 to get towed to Three Rivers.

Don't hate the humble marmot. It's a brave little rodent. With hair standing on end and long claws at the ready, the feisty marmot clatters its sharp teeth and whistles loudly at enemies. Marmots are superbly adapted to survive in a harsh environment. Their bodies afford "clear and cogent arguments of the wisdom and design of the Author" (Robert Boyle, 1688). And, it's against federal law to use poison or other substances to kill, deter, or otherwise foil marmots from car-gnawing.

Remember to get supplies in Three Rivers. Put drinks in a gunnysack and store them in the Kaweah River. That'll chill the cans.

Think about using the walk-in campsites at Cold Springs, nestled in a corner between the Kaweah River and a waterfall that pours down to the river. To access the walk-ins, take the second right loop and follow it to the parking lot at the end. Bring rucksacks to carry your stuff the hundred yards or so into the sites. There is piped water and a pit toilet in among the sites.

A trail (3 miles round-trip) heading east from Cold Springs Campground (trailhead between sites 6 and 7) directs you along a signed nature trail. I found out that corn lilies are also called skunk cabbage and that juniper seeds need to be partially digested by birds in order to sprout, which means they grow far away from their parent trees. Stay on the trail, which travels alongside the Kaweah River, and after roughly 1 mile you'll arrive at the Mineral King picnic area and the neighboring White Chief and Eagle Lake Trailheads, where you can explore more ambitious hiking options.

Plan on spending more than a day or so in the Mineral King Valley. You could spend most of the summer hiking out of Cold Springs Campground, but give yourself a day or two to get used to the altitude.

Cold Springs Campground

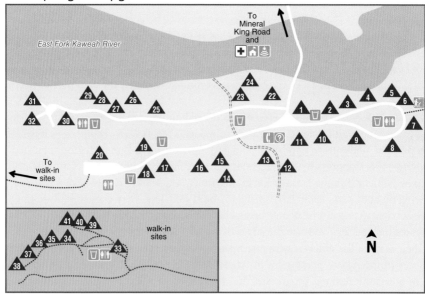

GETTING THERE

From Los Angeles, take I-5 north over the Tejon Pass to CA 99. Take CA 65 north to Exeter. Turn right (east) on CA 198 to Three Rivers. Three miles past Three Rivers turn right onto Mineral King Road. It's about 23 miles to Cold Springs Campground. Plan on the 23-mile trip taking 1.5 hours.

GPS COORDINATES: N36° 27' 05" W118° 36' 41"

24

Dorst Creek Campground

Beauty ★★★★ / Privacy ★★★ / Spaciousness ★★★★ / Quiet ★★★★ / Security ★★★★ / Cleanliness ★★★★★

This is a good summer family campground with wonderful side trips.

Dorst Creek Campground is all about family. On arrival you'll notice squads of children splashing in the nonthreatening Dorst Creek or racing up and down the grassy slopes, as well as moms pushing their infants around in strollers. Most of the folks are tent campers laagered together in the tent-only loops, and their children quickly become friends. I saw lots of dads relaxing in lawn chairs, free and happy.

On the Generals Highway, Dorst Creek Campground is a perfect base camp from which to explore Giant Forest, Grant Grove, and, farther afield, Cedar Grove. Not too far away is Hume Lake, with big-time swimming prospects. A quick run will get you groceries at Lodgepole or Stony Creek Lodge.

An early explorer of what is now Sequoia National Park, William Brewer, wrote: "Such a landscape! A hundred peaks in sight over 13,000 feet—many very sharp, deep canyons, cliffs in every direction almost rivaling Yosemite, sharp ridges almost inaccessible to man, on which human foot has never trod—all combined to produce a view the sublimity of which is rarely equaled, one which few are privileged to behold."

To help you gain a sense of the Giant Forest's scale, note that the pine tree in the center of the photo is 40 feet tall. A shuttle travels between the campground and the Giant Forest Memorial Day–Labor Day.

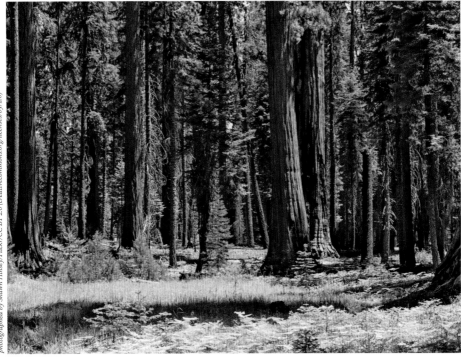

photographed by Shawn Hinsey/Flickr/CC BY 2.0 (creativecommons.org/licenses/by/2.0)

KEY INFORMATION

LOCATION: Sequoia & Kings Canyon National Parks, 10 miles north of the Giant Forest on Generals Highway, Three Rivers, CA 93271

CONTACT: 559-565-3341, nps.gov/seki

OPERATED BY: National Park Service

OPEN: June–September (depending on road and snow conditions)

SITES: 218

EACH SITE: Picnic table, fire ring, bear box

ASSIGNMENT: Site-specific reservations accepted; reservations recommended

REGISTRATION: At entrance or reserve at recreation.gov or 877-444-6777

FACILITIES: Water, flush toilets, wheelchair-accessible sites

PARKING: At site

FEE: $22 plus $9 nonrefundable reservation fee

ELEVATION: 6,700'

RESTRICTIONS:

PETS: On leash only

FIRES: In fire pits; fires may be prohibited during high fire danger

ALCOHOL: No restrictions

VEHICLES: 1 per site; maximum 6 people per site

OTHER: Keep food in bear boxes, not in tents or cars; 14-day stay limit

---

The National Park Service has fought hard to keep it that way. In fact, one of their biggest fights was against sheep. The mountains were perfect for sheepherding. The sheep ran amok through the forests, eating everything in sight, ripping it all up by the roots. Kings Canyon was fast becoming a high-altitude desert. The park superintendent called out the U.S. Cavalry, and still the sheep and shepherds kept coming. Only when the superintendent hit on the strategy of banning sheep on one side of the Sierras and shepherds on the other side was the ovine feeding frenzy discouraged.

A great hike from Dorst Creek Campground leads to the Muir Grove of giant sequoias. Even if you poke along, the round-trip shouldn't take more than 4 hours. Find the trailhead at the Dorst Creek Campground amphitheater (follow the beehive symbol west). The trail is signed and leads you up through white firs and sugar pines, then over a ridge to the Muir Grove giants. The good news is that the return trip is mostly downhill.

Another nearby hike is up Little Baldy. The trailhead is 1.6 miles south of the Dorst Creek Campground entrance on the Generals Highway. Park in the pull-off area at the Little Baldy Saddle and head northeast. Two hard miles later you're on the bare granite Little Baldy summit. It's not a great place to be in a thunderstorm, but it's fine for lying in the noon sun.

If you tire of Dorst Creek Campground family fun, or if you arrive and the campground is full, an alternative lies in the neighboring Sierra National Forest. Leave Dorst Creek Campground and turn left up the Generals Highway toward Grant Grove. Turn right on Big Meadow Road and drive about 5 miles to Big Meadows Campground Number 3. Pass up the heavily used Big Meadows Campground Numbers 1 and 2. Below Number 3, Boulder Creek spills down rocky chutes and gathers in pools. There is good dipping there, but be careful. The rock is slippery.

Or, pick up a fire permit as you pass the Hume Lake Forest Service Station on CA 180, and you can camp in one of literally thousands of wonderful, potential sites for hunkering down overnight.

Farther down the white-knuckle Big Meadow Road is Horse Corral Meadow, where, in 1922, a cowpoke named Jessie Agnew killed the last grizzly bear in California, claiming it was after his cattle. Imagine, killing the last California grizzly, our state animal!

Back at Big Meadows Campground, look for a brown, fiberglass post marking a trailhead. From here, you can hike up to Weaver Lake or Jennie Lake. Take the trail about 2 miles to Fox Meadow where there's a small wooden sign and a trail register. Weaver Lake is straight ahead about 1.5 miles. The trail to Jennie Lake, to the right, heads south 5 miles.

The best way into Dorst Creek Campground is up CA 180 from Fresno. The other road in, through Three Rivers, is a bear. It's narrow, slow, and scary. When you arrive at Dorst Creek Campground, check out all the loops. I camped in a loop allowing trailers and found the campsite much roomier and more private than the sites on the tent-only loops.

Try to camp at Dorst long enough to relax and get to know the area. I think three days is a minimum. One day just doesn't get it. Camping has its own clock, and it runs slowly.

Dorst Creek Campground

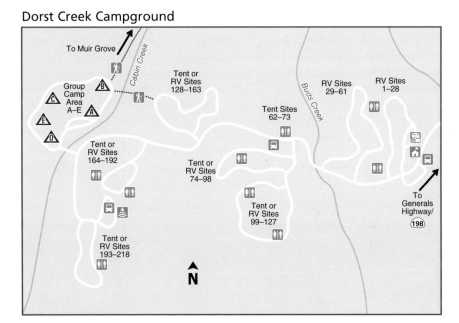

GETTING THERE

From Los Angeles, take I-5 north over the Tejon Pass to CA 99. Drive north on CA 99 to Fresno. Turn right on CA 198 and drive to Kings Canyon National Park. Turn right (south) on the Generals Highway and drive 16 miles to Dorst Creek Campground on the right.

GPS COORDINATES: N36° 38' 10" W118 ° 48' 41"

25

East Fork Campground

Beauty ★★★★★ / Privacy ★★★★★ / Spaciousness ★★★ / Quiet ★★★ / Security ★★★★★ / Cleanliness ★★★★★

Some say East Fork features the best camping in the Sierras.

Going from Los Angeles to East Fork, you'll go through the town of Mojave, the desert, and then the Owens Valley, a 100-mile-long, 5-mile-wide trench—or graben, as geologists call lowlands bounded by faults—between the Sierras on the west and the White-Inyo Mountains on the east. It's a magical place, and the American Indians coined the name Inyo, meaning "dwelling place of the great spirit."

It is a land of dramatic contrast and incredible beauty, where mountain and desert meld into breathtaking scenery, and glaciered peaks tower over shimmering alkali flats. Tumbling mountain streams become lost in the desert, and gemlike lakes shimmer against deep pine forests.

East Fork Campground lies in the heart of Rock Creek, a glacial cirque (basin) that drops 6,000 feet and 20 miles to the Owens River. On the way to East Fork, you'll pass Bishop (the last good town for shopping); don't forget to stop at Mahogany Smoked Meats on US 395 as you leave town. Buy some smoked pork chops for that night's dinner. Gnaw on some world-famous slab jerky as you drive up the infamous Sherwin Grade (or Vaporlock Grade as the old-timers called it). You'll climb 24 miles and about 3,000 feet to Tom's Place Resort, where you will turn south on Rock Creek Road.

Stop at Tom's Place Resort. It's a restaurant/store/bar/cabin complex where you can get fishing information and the bait that the trout are hitting that day. You can buy last-minute

The aptly named Rock Creek travels right beside the East Fork Campground.

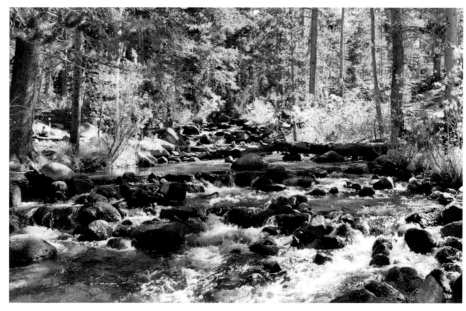

photographed by Marc Mosko

KEY INFORMATION

LOCATION: Rock Creek Road, Mammoth Lakes, CA 93546

CONTACT: 760-873-2400, www.fs.usda.gov/inyo

OPERATED BY: U.S. Forest Service

OPEN: May–November

SITES: 133

EACH SITE: Picnic table, fire ring, food-storage locker

ASSIGNMENT: Some sites require reservations; others are first come, first served

REGISTRATION: At entrance or reserve at recreation.gov or 877-444-6777

FACILITIES: Water, pit toilets

PARKING: At site

FEE: $25

ELEVATION: 9,000'

RESTRICTIONS:

PETS: Allowed

FIRES: In fire pit

ALCOHOL: No restrictions

VEHICLES: RVs up to 22 feet

OTHER: 14-day stay limit

---

camping supplies or eat some of the gut-plug pancakes for breakfast or gravy-soaked chicken fried steak for dinner.

Head up Rock Creek Road past French Camp Campground, a lovely campground by the creek that's almost 1,500 feet lower than East Fork Campground, which makes it a good place to camp in the spring, when the flowers are out down below and East Fork is still socked in with winter cold. At East Fork Campground the bloom arrives later in the summer.

As Owens Valley writer Mary Austin observed, "Well up from the valley, at the confluence of canyons, are delectable summer meadows. Fireweed flames about them against gray boulders; streams are open, go smoothly about the glacier slips, and make deep bluish pools for trout. Pines raise statelier shafts and give themselves room to grow gentians, shinleaf, and little grass of Parnassus in their golden checkered shadows; the meadow is white with violets, and all outdoors keeps the clock."

Find the entrance to East Fork Campground at about 9,000 feet (auto parts stores often sell car altimeters for less than $20, which are surprisingly accurate and fun to watch). The campground is down on Rock Creek. Most of the sites on the creek are lovely but in the open, with RV-size parking spots. Other sites, back up from the creek, are small and private. The parking spots are half a dozen yards from the campsites, which are mostly private and secluded in little copses of pine, brush, and aspen.

When I was there in late September, the aspen leaves were turning gold. When the wind blew they shimmered so prettily in the sunlight and made a soft, tinny clatter as they shook. The creek was well stocked. Happy fishermen tromped back to their campfires with strings of nice-sized trout for dinner. At night, the cold snapped, and in the morning our camping neighbors all exclaimed how nippy it was.

The hardy ridges above the riparian campground are covered with isolated foxtail pines. The creek goes north and south, so the sun is quick to set at night and slow to rise in the morning. At 9,000 feet, you really want the sun and will walk with your morning coffee to find it. A nice evening walk is across the bridges to the other side of the creek. Go to site 108, the host's site, and across the access road you'll find the first bridge. There is fine fishing here.

A solid hike is up the creek to Rock Creek Lake. The trail leaves on the north side of the campground by site 82 and goes all the way to Rock Creek Lake, passing some small campgrounds and a resort before hitting the lake and trailheads to the high country.

Above Rock Creek Lake, you'll find Mosquito Flat. You can drive there and park at 10,250 feet. From there, it's an easy day hike into the John Muir Wilderness and Little Lakes Valley. The valley is a pretty glacial trough below 13,000-foot peaks. Bring your wildflower book because the meadows up there are loaded with wildflowers.

East Fork Campground

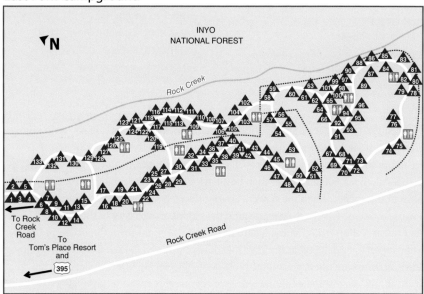

GETTING THERE

From Los Angeles, take I-5 north about 24 miles to Exit 162/CA 14. Take CA 14 north about 118 miles to US 395 near Inyokern. Continue north on US 395 about 127 miles to Bishop. From Bishop, drive 24 miles north on US 395 and exit to the west at Tom's Place Resort onto Rock Creek Road. Drive 5 miles up Rock Creek Road to the campground.

GPS COORDINATES: N37° 29' 01" W118° 43' 07"

26

Fairview Campground

Beauty ★★★★★ / Privacy ★★★★ / Spaciousness ★★★★ / Quiet ★★★★ / Security ★★★★ / Cleanliness ★★★★

Fairview Campground offers the best tent camping in the Lake Isabella area.

About 60,000 years ago, a glacier flowing down an earthquake slip fault cut the U-shaped Upper Kern Canyon. Look southward along the Upper Kern Canyon and you can see how the glacier carved out the canyon, giving it rounded shoulders. In the Lower Kern Canyon, below Lake Isabella, where the glacier didn't flow, the shoulders of the canyon are sharp and V-shaped.

Fairview Campground, near the head of the Upper Kern Valley, is the best camping spot in the area. It's set down by the river, well below the road and any traffic noise, with the mountains towering around. The sites are so well planned it's hard to decide where to camp. The last time I was there it was spring, and the snow level was down to 5,000 feet, but it was warm and sunny down in the campground.

All the flowers were out—most ostentatiously the purple yerba santa. We made a tea out of its leaves, which American Indians thought was good for coughs, colds, asthma, and the like. Pretty bitter stuff. I've also heard that the leaves, when pounded into a poultice, cure sores. The Spanish used the leaves as tobacco, for chewing and smoking. Others claim that you can chew the leaves to quench thirst. After the first bitter taste subsides, you'll feel a sweet, cooling sensation. I tried it, and it wasn't too bad.

Once you visit the high desert of the Upper Kern Valley, you'll be hooked.

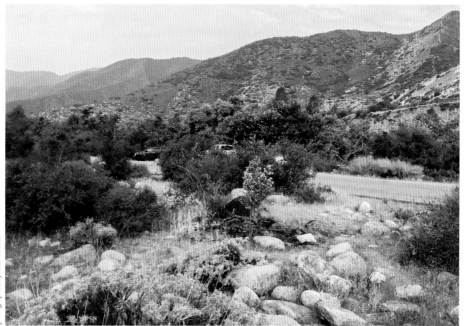

photographed by Adam Reeder

KEY INFORMATION

LOCATION: 1941 Kern River Hwy.,
Kernville, CA 93238

CONTACT: 559-784-1500,
www.fs.usda.gov/sequoia

OPERATED BY: U.S. Forest Service

OPEN: April–November

SITES: 55

EACH SITE: Picnic table, fire ring

ASSIGNMENT: Reservations recommended

REGISTRATION: Host collects on rounds;
reserve (at least 3 days in advance) at
recreation.gov or 877-444-6777

FACILITIES: Water, vault toilets,
wheelchair-accessible sites

PARKING: At site

FEE: $25–$27 plus $9 nonrefundable
reservation fee

ELEVATION: 3,500'

RESTRICTIONS:

PETS: On leash only

FIRES: In fire pit

ALCOHOL: No restrictions

VEHICLES: RVs up to 45 feet

By our campsite, we found a flowering flannel bush (*Fremontia californica*) with brazen yellow flowers bright against the white water of the Kern. All night, the strong current rattled the rocks on the river bottom. In the morning, the ranger, who came by to collect our fee, admired our flannel bush and reported that the bark can be brewed and gargled to relieve a sore throat.

Fairview has always been blessed. American Indians used it as a fall and spring campground. In the late 1800s, Stony Rhymes and Lucien Barbeau had a cow camp on the bend of the river. In 1910, Matt and Lupe Burlando moved to Fairview and built the Fairview Lodge. They rented rooms to tourists who came for fishing and hunting. Matt built a swinging bridge (you can still see it today) across the river to the natural hot springs on the west side and ran packing trips into the backcountry. After Matt and Lupe's children reached school age, the entire family moved down to Kernville to be near the school. Fairview went back to being a cow camp for a while before Johnny McNally opened McNally's Steakhouse. Johnny was an amazing rodeo rider and a deputy sheriff, and his wife, Pauline, could shoot a running buck with a rifle from the back of a galloping horse.

To reach McNally's from the campground, walk south along the river 50 yards. You'll find McNally's Steakhouse, the hamburger hut, and the gas station/grocery store. We loaded up on beer, hot dogs, and ice at the store and then hunkered down at the outside picnic tables for some rousing chiliburgers before heading across the suspension bridge on a diet-redeeming hike along Flynn Trail. (See the map and handout sheet on the display by the parking lot near the hamburger stand.) You'll find access here for the Tobias Trail as well. Maybe the best short day hikes here are on the Whiskey Flat Trail, which runs from the bridge down to the north end of Burlando Road in Kernville. The trail parallels the west side of the river and runs through high chaparral, digger pines, and oak. There are wonderful places along the trail for picnicking. Put down a blanket and snooze while the river runs below you. I've heard there's good fishing here. Another good hike is up the trail to Salmon Creek Falls. The marked trailhead is a mile or so south of Fairview to the east.

One word of warning about the Kern River: it is very dangerous. When I was last there in May, it was running way above its natural banks. Camping there with children is only advisable if they are sternly warned and constantly watched. The water is cold, and the current is strong. If you're camping with children, go down below to Isabella Lake. I especially recommend Tillie Creek Campground, which is pretty, safe, and flat. Bring the children's bicycles. There is even a playground. In the spring, good fishing can be found in the lake as well.

Fairview Campground

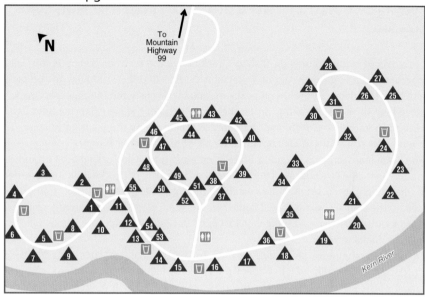

GETTING THERE

From Los Angeles, take I-5 north to CA 99 past Bakersfield. Take CA 178 east to Lake Isabella. Take CA 155 north to Wofford Heights. Bear right to Kernville. From Kernville, drive north 16 miles on Sierra Way/Mountain Highway 99 to Fairview Campground on the left.

GPS COORDINATES: N35° 55' 44" W118° 29' 30"

27

Four Jeffrey and Sabrina Campgrounds

Beauty ★★★★ / Privacy ★★★★ / Spaciousness ★★★★★ / Quiet ★★★★★ / Security ★★★★★ / Cleanliness ★★★★★

Four Jeffrey Campground is the best destination campground in the Bishop Creek drainage area.

The princess of campgrounds on Bishop Creek above the town of Bishop is tiny Sabrina Campground perched on the lip of Lake Sabrina. At 9,000 feet, the view of the picture-perfect lake, the glaciered mountain peaks marbled with rusty red metamorphic rock, and the deep blue sky is breathtaking. Sit on the sunny patio of the Lake Sabrina Boat Landing and eat an incredible old-fashioned hamburger grilled up by the pleasant hostess. That's how you know you're not in Switzerland after all, but in the Wild West.

You'll see lanky anglers swigging Budweiser, a big husky dog asleep atop an upturned aluminum boat, and cowpokes in 10-gallon hats stepping out of canoes, holding up 6-pound trout, just caught, their bright colors catching the sun. Then, oddly, a pack train of llamas will file up the trail across the lake. Llamas? In the Wild West? Yes, apparently some of the local pack outfits use llamas. Indigenous to Peruvian high country, the llamas take to the Sierras like ducks to water.

Drive the vertiginous, short dirt road up to North Lake and check out North Lake Campground at the trailhead. No trailers, no RVs, only tents, but like Sabrina Campground and most of the campgrounds in the Bishop Creek area, it has few sites. The only campground around that has enough space to be a destination campground is Four Jeffrey, which is down the road from Sabrina Lake and to the right, on the spur road to South Lake.

The South and Middle Forks of Bishop Creek converge near Four Jeffrey Campground.

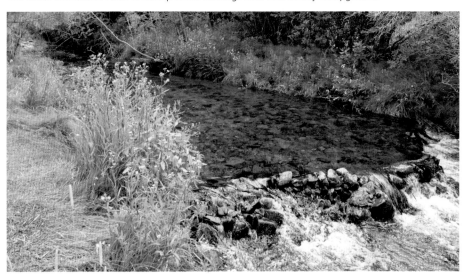

photographed by Dharam Kaur Khalsa

KEY INFORMATION

LOCATION: Four Jeffrey Campground:
S. Lake Road, Bishop, CA 93514

CONTACT: 760-873-2400,
www.fs.usda.gov/inyo

OPERATED BY: U.S. Forest Service

OPEN: Four Jeffrey, April 26–October 29;
Sabrina, May 15–October 15

SITES: Four Jeffrey 106, Sabrina 20

EACH SITE: Picnic table, fire ring

ASSIGNMENT: First come, first served;
no reservations (Sabrina); reservations
recommended (Four Jeffrey)

REGISTRATION: At entrance (Sabrina);
reserve (at least 4 days in advance) at recre
ation.gov or 877-444-6777 (Four Jeffrey)

FACILITIES: Water, flush toilets,
wheelchair-accessible sites

PARKING: At site

FEE: $26 (Sabrina); $26 plus $9 nonrefund-
able reservation fee (Four Jeffrey)

ELEVATION: 8,100'

RESTRICTIONS:

PETS: On leash only

FIRES: In fire pit

ALCOHOL: No restrictions

VEHICLES: RVs up to 22 feet

OTHER: Four Jeffrey, 14-day stay limit;
Sabrina, 7-day stay limit

Four Jeffrey is an impressive campground. The surrounding mountains are spare and dry, and the view is incredible, although not eye-poppingly stunning like the views from Sabrina and North Lake. The South Fork of Bishop Creek runs through the campground. Many of the sites are down by the water, which is alive with trout. Others are up the hill in low brush. This area makes for good spring and early-summer camping. By fall, the hillside is muted and austere. I like that look, but others may want the green of the pines.

Make Four Jeffrey the first-night destination campground in the Bishop Creek area. Chances of getting a site there are very good (the camping season at Four Jeffrey is two months longer than at Sabrina Campground). The next day, cruise around. Hit Sabrina Campground first, then North Lake Campground, then the other little campgrounds up and down the forks of Bishop Creek, and see if you find something you like better.

Part of my attraction to Four Jeffrey Campground has to do with survival. All the other campgrounds except little North Lake are by the streambed. And, the Bishop area is earth-quake country. At 2:30 a.m. in March 1872, a monster quake hit the Owens Valley. It was felt as far east as Salt Lake City, as far north as Canada, and as far south as Mexico. It shook John Muir over in Yosemite Valley. He described the incident: "I was awakened by a tremendous earthquake, and though I had never enjoyed a storm of this sort, the strange thrilling motion could not be mistaken, and I ran out of my cabin, both glad and frightened, shouting, 'A noble earthquake! A noble earthquake!' feeling sure I was going to learn something."

I figure a quake like that could happen again, and the dams up on Sabrina and South Lake might possibly go pretty easily. I want to be sleeping on the high ground at Four Jeffrey Campground, so I can snooze right through the flood.

The best shopping is down the road in Bishop. The road in and out is good and fast. Bishop (named for Samuel A. Bishop, one of the area's original cattle ranchers) is a cow town recently encased in an ugly, fat pocket of fast-food franchises. Fortunately, Schat's Dutch Bakery is there for sheepherder bread; Jack's Waffle Shop is open for breakfast with locals and cowpokes; the Firehouse Grill still attracts tourists; and Mahogany Smoked

Meats (north on US 395) still sells various varieties of mahogany-smoked jerky so you can gnaw your merry way through the High Sierras.

Four Jeffrey Campground

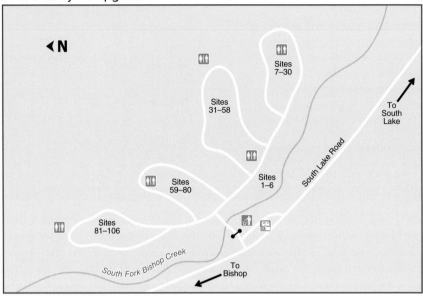

Sabrina Campground

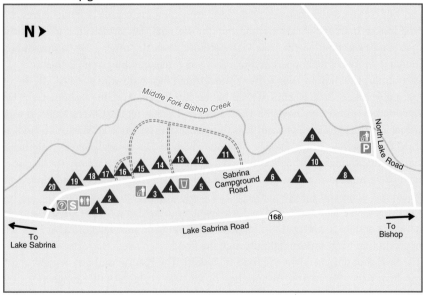

GETTING THERE

From Los Angeles, take I-5 north to CA 14 to US 395 near Inyokern. Continue north on US 395 for 123 miles to Bishop. Drive 13 miles south on CA 168 to S. Lake Road. Go left for a mile or so to Four Jeffrey Campground. Sabrina Campground is another 4 miles south on CA 168 from that turnoff.

GPS COORDINATES: N37° 14' 56" W118° 34' 14"

Four Jeffrey Campground typically opens just in time for fishing season.

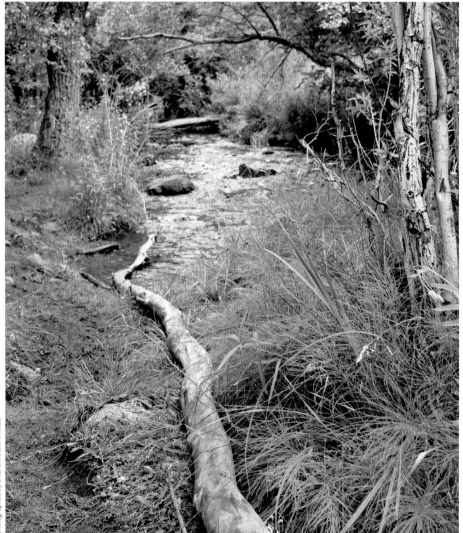

photographed by Dharam Kaur Khalsa

28

Horse Meadow Campground

Beauty ★★★★★ / Privacy ★★ / Spaciousness ★★★ / Quiet ★★★★ / Security ★★★ / Cleanliness ★★★★

This is my favorite tent campground. It's difficult to get up here, but it's worth it for the beauty and solitude.

Horse Meadow Campground is my favorite campground. I don't even know why. Maybe it's the long grind up the mountains, or the terrain—that dry, big-sky country look with the pines, boulders, and open green meadows. Maybe I watched too many Westerns when I was a child. The sky at Horse Meadow Campground just seems a little bit bluer.

The campsites at Horse Meadow are roomy and offer a great view. Salmon Creek runs through the campground and gurgles just enough to lull you to sleep. Below the meadow, it gathers in pools deep enough for you to take a freezing dip. When you hop out, warm yourself on the hot granite slabs.

Getting to Horse Meadow is part of the fun. Pass McNally's Hamburger Stand near Fairview Campground (see page 87) on your way north of Kernville. You're into the wilderness now, so stock up while you can. Here, the canyon narrows, and you see cliffs of metamorphic rock colored by chartreuse lichen. Notice the tailings from Fairview Mine across the river. This is gold country. Pass Lower Campground and Fairview Campground, and soon enough you turn right on Sherman Pass Road.

In the early 1860s William H. Brewer explored the Greenhorn Mountains as part of the California Geologic Survey; today, you can view them from a trail near Horse Meadow Campground.

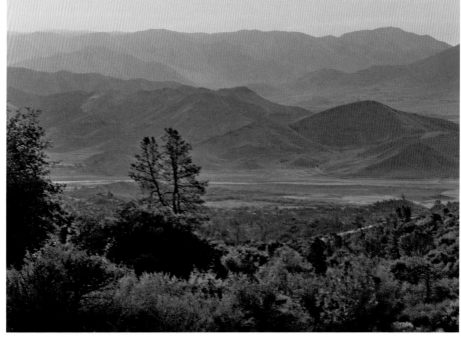

photographed by Tom Hilton/Flickr/CC BY 2.0 (creativecommons.org/licenses/by/2.0)

KEY INFORMATION

LOCATION: FS 22S12, Kernville, CA 93238

CONTACT: 559-784-1500,
www.fs.usda.gov/sequoia

OPERATED BY: U.S. Forest Service

OPEN: Memorial Day–mid-October

SITES: 41 total; 26 for tents;
15 for RVs up to 22 feet long

EACH SITE: Picnic table, fire ring

ASSIGNMENT: First come, first served;
no reservations

REGISTRATION: At entrance

FACILITIES: Vault toilets, water
(phone ahead to make sure)

PARKING: At site

FEE: $17

ELEVATION: 7,600'

RESTRICTIONS:

PETS: On leash only

FIRES: In fire pits

ALCOHOL: No restrictions

VEHICLES: Trailers not recommended

Sherman Pass Road heads up past buck brush, mountain mahogany, and fremontia, into chaparral with gray and pinyon pine, and finally, into Jeffrey pine, black oak, cedar, and white fir as you turn right on Cherry Hill Road. It's about 10 miles up to Horse Meadow Campground, past Alder and Brush Creeks, then Poison Meadow (note the dispersed camping sites, which require a fire permit). At the junction with Horse Meadow Road, go right 1.3 miles and you're in a tent-camping paradise.

The campground has two loops. The right loop is for tent camping only and runs along a hill above Salmon Creek and the meadow. The left loop is for tenters and small RVs. The last time I was there in July, most of the folks were tent campers. The narrow ascents up Sherman Pass and Cherry Hill Roads deter RVs and trailers. And, once you're up here, it's a long, long way down for supplies. There is good water (phone the ranger station before coming to make sure), but no trash bins. Haul out your garbage.

Horse Meadow is a good place to bring children. The campground loops are fine for biking, and Salmon Creek offers good trout fishing, but it's not wild and dangerous like the Kern. There are many easy hikes around the meadow, including several along Salmon Creek to some good dipping pools.

To find the upper bathing pools, go to the south side of the Horse Meadow Campground's main loop and find the trail that parallels the creek. Walk east along the left bank of the creek. Cross a spur road over Salmon Creek and keep climbing, follow the creek, and you'll come to the pools.

To visit the downstream pools, walk back past the camp entrance and go left down Salmon Falls Trail. Follow the signed trail from the parking lot and skirt the meadow. When the trail crosses Salmon Creek on a big log and goes left around a rocky butte, don't follow it. Instead, head west down the right side of the creek. The trail meanders along over rocky areas, bypassing clumps of willows, and leads you past some prime pools for dipping. The water is frigid, but the sun is blazing hot. This is heaven!

For a major hike, go back to the big log that crosses over Salmon Creek. With a backpack filled with drinks and sandwiches, head around the rocky butte toward Salmon Creek Falls. The trail skirts the meadow and then heads into the woods. It crosses canyons while following the south side of Salmon Creek through purple lupine country with monks hood, larkspur, and red bugler. Down by the creek, you'll see willows and dogwood.

The trail continues down to the north side of Salmon Creek and ends with a view of the Greenhorn Mountains. Those more agile than me can rock-hop down to the creek, where there are more wonderful pools for bathing. Just beyond them, you'll find the top of Salmon Creek Falls.

Horse Meadow Campground

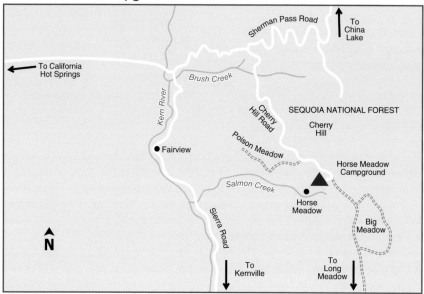

GETTING THERE

From Los Angeles, take I-5 north to CA 99. Pass Bakersfield and take CA 178 east to Lake Isabella. Take CA 155 to Wofford Heights. Bear right to Kernville. Drive north on Sierra Way 19.4 miles and turn right on Sherman Pass Road, signed HIGHWAY 395—BLACK ROCK RANGER STATION. Drive 6 miles, turn right on Cherry Hill Road, signed HORSE MEADOW—BIG MEADOW. Drive 9.1 miles on the (sometimes dirt) road to the signed campground-entrance road on the right.

GPS COORDINATES: N35° 54' 05.9" W118° 22' 20.8"

29

Kern Plateau Dispersed Camping Area

Beauty ★★★★★ / Privacy ★★★★★ / Spaciousness ★★★★★ / Quiet ★★★★★ / Security ★ / Cleanliness ★★★★★

Set on a high-elevation Sierra plateau, this loosely defined area offers an unstructured, open camping experience, free of charge, no reservations needed.

For many, the open camping experience of the Kern Plateau is tent camping as it should be, especially for hunters, anglers, hikers, 4x4 enthusiasts, and off-road motorcyclists. Most often referred to as Kennedy Meadows, this unspoiled high-sierra plateau boasts acres of granite outcroppings, tall redwood trees, and pristine green meadows. Think of it as Yosemite Valley without the excess bureaucracy. It should be noted that there are formal, maintained campgrounds located in the area with facilities—Kennedy Meadows, Troy Meadow, Horse Meadow, and Fish Creek Campgrounds—but that's not what this is all about. For more information on these campgrounds, visit the U.S. Forest Service website at www.fs.usda.gov/sequoia.

The Kern Plateau is one of the rare places in the Sierra Nevada Mountain range where you can still hunt, fish, drive 4x4 vehicles, and ride OHVs legally. Though legal, these activities are regulated, and self-policed by users. You cannot simply go off-roading anywhere, only on marked trails and roads, and if you act like a goon, expect to be called out. A dedicated community of enthusiasts maintains the trails and roads, so it's not a place to go tear it up. Because it is well respected by users, the Kern Plateau area is pristine, despite the presence of what some deem destructive outdoor activities.

Uncommonly scenic views are commonplace on the Kern Plateau.

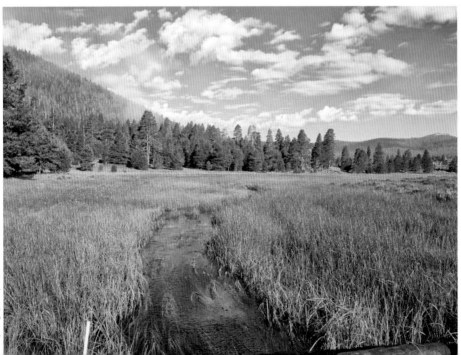

photographed by Charles Patterson

KEY INFORMATION

LOCATION: FS 22S05, Inyokern, CA 93527

CONTACT: 760-873-2400,
www.fs.usda.gov/sequoia

OPERATED BY: U.S. Forest Service

OPEN: Summer

SITES: Open area

EACH SITE: No amenities

ASSIGNMENT: First come, first served;
no reservations

REGISTRATION: Not required

FACILITIES: None

PARKING: Some pullouts; otherwise, less than
10 feet off established dirt roads

FEE: None

ELEVATION: 7,000'–9,000'

RESTRICTIONS:

PETS: On leash only

FIRES: In fire rings

ALCOHOL: No restrictions

VEHICLES: Trailers not recommended

The main appeal of this area for anyone visiting is the ability to find your own campsite, with nobody around and nothing but backwoods solitude. To find a place to camp, you may simply explore any of the marked dirt roads that branch off FS 22S05, or Sherman Pass Road. Unless otherwise marked, the campsites are all fair game. You can also check out some of the more popular areas: Troy Meadow Overflow, Fish Creek Overflow, Bonita Meadow, and the South Fork of the Kern River around Kennedy Meadows, as well as Big Meadow and Osa and Paloma Meadows. Some sites will even have fire rings. Remember, before lighting any campfire, you must acquire a campfire permit, and consult with rangers about fire risk. The Kern Plateau is a gem—it would be a shame to see it go up in smoke (cue Smokey Bear).

Although it's a treat for almost every type of outdoor person, the Kern Plateau is perhaps most ideal for off-road motorcyclists. That's because there are hundreds of miles of idyllic singletrack trails that are maintained and mapped by the motorcycle clubs that frequent the area. They're even rated for technical difficulty, and several sections are designated one-way travel only. It's worth noting that the Kern Plateau isn't ideal for novice or young beginner riders, who should search elsewhere for more open, less difficult terrain. For an online listing of OHV trails, visit the U.S. Forest Service website at www.fs.usda.gov/activity/sequoia/recreation/ohv/?recid=79563&actid=93. It's strongly recommended that before you explore any of this terrain, acquire detailed topographic maps and carry a handheld GPS or smartphone to keep your bearings.

If you're a hiker, don't let the presence of motorcycles scare you off. The motorcycle trails are multiuse, which means you're a welcomed visitor too. Hikers often report seeing few motorcycles, if any at all, and are surprised at the pristine condition of the trails and the politeness of encountered motorcyclists. If you really want to go off the beaten path, however, the neighboring Domeland Wilderness and nearby Pacific Crest Trail are off limits to motorized vehicles, so you can really enjoy the silence.

Do not get so caught up in the magic of Kern Plateau that you forget about safety. Kern Plateau is bear country. Black bears are all over the place, and some of them so are so large, you'll swear you saw a grizzly. Though extremely people-shy, black bears have the potential to be dangerous in rare circumstances, so always observe standard bear safety protocol. There are no serious weather considerations for this entire area because it's essentially off-limits in fall, winter, and spring, when the road shuts down due to snowfall. However, visitors should always understand that High Sierra weather can be unpredictable. Below-freezing nighttime temps, snow showers, hail storms, heavy downpours, and lightning storms can happen without warning—so camp accordingly.

The Kern Plateau is perhaps summed up best as the un-Yosemite. There are no exorbitant fees, nor are there crowds of tourists, smog, tour buses, and traffic. It's a place that can be enjoyed by everyone, which is why everyone should give it the utmost respect. Clean up after yourself, respect the environment, and be nice to other visitors.

Kern Plateau Dispersed Camping Area

GETTING THERE

There are two ways into the Kern Plateau area—from the eastern side of the Sierras, and from the west. From the Eastern Sierra, head north from the town of Pearsonville on US 395 and turn left on 9 Mile Canyon Road. For approximately 25 miles, ascend the steep, winding road, which will become Kennedy Meadow Road and then Sherman Pass Road. From the western side of the Sierras, make your way to Bakersfield and CA 178. Follow this treacherous highway to Lake Isabella, and after approximately 67 miles turn left on Chimney Peak Road for a little over 12 miles and stay left on Chimney Basin Road, then, after 2.2 miles, turn left on Kennedy Meadow Road/Sherman Pass Road/FS 22S05. After roughly 13 miles you'll have entered the Kern Plateau area.

GPS COORDINATES: N36° 01' 22" W118° 08' 09"

30

Lower Peppermint Campground

Beauty ★★★★ / Privacy ★★★★ / Spaciousness ★★★★ / Quiet ★★★★★ / Security ★★★★ / Cleanliness ★★★★★

The Lower Peppermint area is astonishingly beautiful, with waterslides, waterfalls, and mountain peaks.

Lower Peppermint sits smack dab in the middle of great Northern Sierra camping near the spectacular scenery of Dome Rock and the Needles. On your way, obtain a California Campfire Permit to increase your camping possibilities a hundredfold. You can get one from Greenhorn Ranger Station on CA 155, at Lake Isabella, a few miles east of Bakersfield, or at Cannell Meadow Ranger Station in Kernville. The free permit allows you to camp almost anywhere in Sequoia National Forest.

Sequoia National Forest calls this dispersed camping, meaning you can camp anywhere not posted off-limits. For example, around Lloyd Meadow Road dozens of old logging roads or turnoffs allow you to drive a few hundred yards and camp in a private area. Of course, you'll be expected to follow the forest's regulations—cart out your garbage, dig catholes for bodily waste, and burn your toilet paper. Try not to leave any traces of your visit.

Buy groceries in Lake Isabella or Kernville—once you get on Lloyd Meadow Road, supplies are limited to the humble inventory of the general store at Johnsondale R-Ranch in the Sequoias (turn off Parker Pass Drive 0.6 mile east of Lloyd Meadow Road). You'll pass a cowboy guard at the gate; tell him you want to shop at the store, and he'll wave you on.

Use your campsite's fire ring to make a large pot of campfire chili.

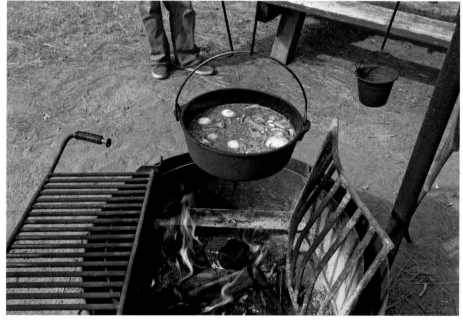

photographed by Hypatia Luna

KEY INFORMATION

LOCATION: FS 22S82, Springville, CA 93265

CONTACT: 559-539-2607 or 559-784-1500, www.fs.usda.gov/sequoia

OPERATED BY: U.S. Forest Service

OPEN: May 15–November 15 (weather permitting)

SITES: 17

EACH SITE: Picnic table, fire ring

ASSIGNMENT: First come, first served; no reservations

REGISTRATION: At entrance

FACILITIES: Vault toilets, water

PARKING: At site

FEE: $17

ELEVATION: 5,300'

RESTRICTIONS:

PETS: Allowed

FIRES: In fire pits

ALCOHOL: No restrictions

VEHICLES: Trailers not recommended

The R-Ranch is a private campground. The lifetime membership fee gives access to cabins, horses, RVs, trails, and more.

Winding Lloyd Meadow Road passes through pine, white fir, cedar, and oak where there is water, and manzanita, fremontia, and digger pine where it's dry. Note turnoffs to the numbered fire safe area camps, which offer good camping (a fire permit is required to camp in fire safe areas, as in all dispersed areas). During dry spells dispersed camping is confined to these areas only.

Lower Peppermint Campground is a small, pretty campground mostly frequented by tent campers. Boy Scouts from nearby Camp Whitsett maintain Lower Peppermint in return for the user fees on their own camp. The sites that adjoin the creek are lovely.

For a great hike and a swim, scramble down the bluff to the foot of the falls. Stop and swim there, or bear left along the creek until you strike a trail that takes you east. It forks south to another area of rocky pools and cascades perfect for picnicking, swimming, and sunbathing.

However, the water runs stronger than it seems, and the wet rocks by the stream are slick. The dry granite slabs above are just as bad. The granite decomposes, and the little dry bits are like ball bearings.

Another good water hike leads to the Alder Slabs. Wear clothes you don't care about, because this trip involves sliding down water chutes into cold pools on your behind. It's fun! Backtrack south on Lloyd Meadow Road and park by gated Sequoia National Forest Route 22S83. Walk north on the dirt road and then turn right down a path to Alder Creek.

Alternately, drive north from Lower Peppermint Campground to see the Needles. These amazing rock formations are crystals formed under pressure from molten rock. Pushed up, the Needles cooled along vertical master joints. Ice and erosion have done the rest. Farther north, see the Freeman Creek Grove of sequoias. En route, investigate the little intersecting roads for good future camping sites. In the dead of summer, you might want to be near water, but in the late spring, this area is so beautiful it doesn't matter where you camp—you'll be blown away by the sight of all the flowers.

Bring a saw for wood gathering, and don't forget a trowel for catholes. I often bring a leaf rake with a sawed-off handle for clearing debris around the picnic tables and fire rings, and a shovel for fire control and digging out if the car gets stuck.

Lower Peppermint Campground

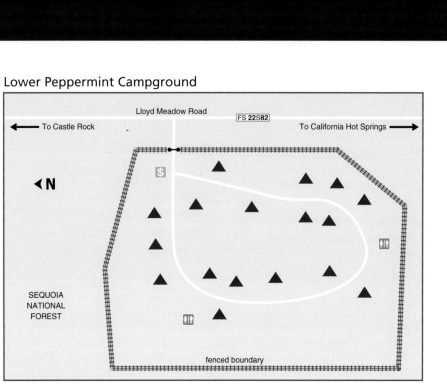

GETTING THERE

From Los Angeles, take I-5 north over the Tejon Pass to CA 99. Drive north on CA 99 past Bakersfield. Take CA 178 east to Lake Isabella. Take CA 155 to Wofford Heights. Bear right to Kernville. From Kernville, drive north on Sierra Way 19.4 miles and turn left on Parker Pass Drive. It is 4.9 miles to the right-hand turn onto Lloyd Meadow Road (FS 22S82). Drive north 13.4 miles to Lower Peppermint Campground. Camp six is a few hundred yards north on the right.

GPS COORDINATES: N36° 03' 59" W118° 29' 27"

31

Minaret Falls Campground

Beauty ★★★★★ / Privacy ★★★ / Spaciousness ★★★★★ / Quiet ★★★★★ / Security ★★★★★ / Cleanliness ★★★★

Check out the prettiest campground in a string of beautiful, popular options on the Upper San Joaquin River west of Mammoth Mountain.

When you drive down the dirt road into the campground, silvery Minaret Falls leaps out at you. Even in late September, on my last visit, the water cascaded down the mountainside like streams of crystal.

Right away, my wife and I drove into a campsite with a clean and soft tent pitch shrouded by trees. Through the willows we could see the riverbank and the falls. We drove a few miles up the road to Red's Meadow Resort & Pack Station to buy worms and salmon eggs for trout fishing. A little bear was raiding the back room of the store, but the clerk and a tourist scared him away. A dog lunged, at the end of his leash, barking at the curious animal as it scurried off. We learned that the original Red was a gold miner who turned to tourism when the Depression and falling gold prices drove him out of business. His pack station at Red's Meadow was one of the first tourist draws in the Mammoth area.

The campground's namesake is the main attraction here.

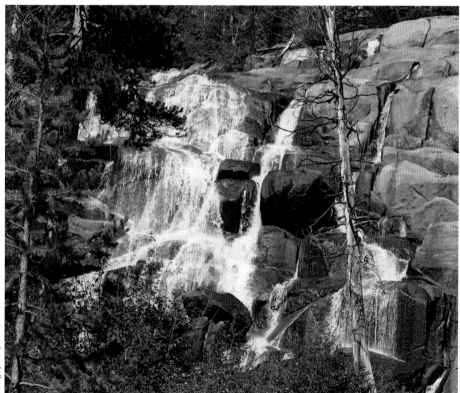

photographed by Rob Gendreau

KEY INFORMATION

LOCATION: Minaret Road,
Mammoth Lakes, CA 93546

CONTACT: 760-924-5500,
www.fs.usda.gov/inyo

OPERATED BY: U.S. Forest Service

OPEN: June 15–September 19

SITES: 27

EACH SITE: Picnic table, fire ring

ASSIGNMENT: First come, first served;
no reservations

REGISTRATION: At entrance

FACILITIES: Water, chemical toilets

PARKING: At site

FEE: $23

ELEVATION: 7,600'

RESTRICTIONS:

PETS: On leash only

FIRES: In fire pit

ALCOHOL: No restrictions

VEHICLES: RVs up to 22 feet

OTHER: No dispersed camping in this area;
14-day stay limit. *Note:* To reduce vehicle
traffic into the Devils Postpile area, a shuttle bus system has been implemented.
Campers pay a one-time exception fee of
$10 per vehicle. Stop at the Mammoth
Lakes visitor center (on the right side of CA
203 on the way into Mammoth Lakes) or
the Adventure Center (at the ski area) for
more information.

We hiked the 1.25 miles down to Rainbow Falls along with a passel of other folks. We took the rough stairs down to the exquisite falls and stood in the spray. A rainbow arced through the mist.

We hiked back through an area of firs, lodgepoles, and Jeffrey pines, scarred like most of Devils Postpile National Monument by a 1992 wildfire. Following the fire, rangers walked through the burn to assess the damage, and charred trees crashed down around them. It wasn't safe to walk there for months.

Back at the Minaret Falls Campground we floated salmon eggs and earthworms down the river and caught six trout. My wife wrapped them in aluminum foil with herbs and cooked them over the campfire. It was a gorgeous night. From the Southern Sierras you can often see hundreds of shooting stars.

Sleeping that night in our tent, I heard the rustle of a visitor—a bear. He ran away when I got up. I inspected the damage. My two treasured inflatable camp sinks, which my wife and I use to wash the dishes, were ruined. The bear had bitten a big hole in each of them. To add insult to injury, he also bit into my plastic collapsible water jug. Were these acts of rancor, or did he think they were full of food?

A neighbor came over. The bear had tried to open the hatch of his Nissan Z; the telltale paw marks gave the intruder away. I told him about my camp sinks. He recommended wiping sinks, picnic tables, and cooler tops each night with bleach. Bears like soap—and everything except bleach. I went back to my sleeping bag and heard the bear slouch through the camp again.

The next morning we walked north along the river and crossed on a log at the end of the campground. There's a short trail to the foot of Minaret Falls. We bushwhacked up to the top of the falls and dipped in some nice pools.

Later, we hiked up to Shadow Lake. It's no easy climb (round-trip is about 7 miles), but you'll agree it's worth it when you see beautiful blue Shadow Lake against huge, craggy Mount Ritter. To find the trailhead, drive back toward Mammoth from the Minaret Falls

Campground. Take the road to Agnew Meadows Campground. About 0.3 mile in, you'll find trailhead parking with toilets and drinking water. Follow the signs to Shadow Lake, through another parking lot and across a creek to another trail junction at about 1 mile. To the left is Red's Meadow. To the right is Shadow Lake. With Mammoth Mountain at your back, climb up past Olaine Lake, cross the San Joaquin River on a wooden bridge, and hoof it up the canyon wall to Shadow Lake. You'll find good fishing, so bring your fishing gear and bait.

Minaret Falls Campground is popular. Be sure to phone rangers ahead of time to make sure it's open and to see how crowded it will be. Try to plan a trip before or after the prime summertime season and arrive on Thursday if you want to spend the weekend. The area is so popular that during the summer, hikers (not campers) are required to park their cars at the Mammoth Ski Resort and take an intra-valley shuttle down.

You have 30 minutes from the time you occupy a campsite to pay. Park your car at the first empty campsite you find and use that 30 minutes to walk around and see if you like another site better. If you find one, leave something on the picnic table and go move your car.

Minaret Falls Campground

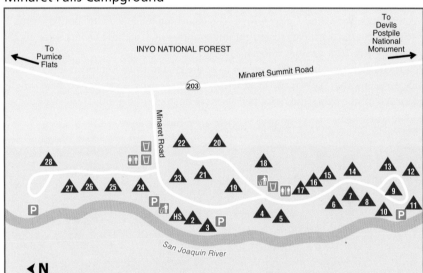

GETTING THERE

From Los Angeles, take I-5 north to CA 14. Take CA 14 north to US 395 near Inyokern. Continue north on US 395 for 123 miles to Bishop. Continue another 37 miles on US 395 to Mammoth Lakes. From Mammoth Lakes, drive 16 miles west on CA 203 (Minaret Summit Road) to the campground.

GPS COORDINATES: N37° 38' 22" W119° 05' 02"

32

⛺ Moraine Campground

Beauty ★★★★★ / Privacy ★★★ / Spaciousness ★★★★ / Quiet ★★★★★ / Security ★★★★ / Cleanliness ★★★★★

A grand canyon and a pretty valley combine for sublime scenery.

Moraine Campground is simply sublime. And it's the mountains—not the standard national park–issue campground—that elicit this feeling. You would not come to Moraine Campground if it were not below Sentinel Ridge and Monarch Divide. However, just the spectacular drive justifies a visit. Take the wide and well-banked, convict-built CA 180 all the way in from Fresno. Coming over the rise to see the gorge and the mountains behind it takes your breath away. Then, circle down and follow the river to Cedar Grove Village and Moraine Campground.

Cedar Grove Market sells ice, beverages, and some food, and there is a cafeteria for folks tired of camp cooking. There are hot showers and a Laundromat. For an ice cream or a sandwich, stop at Kings Canyon Lodge on the way in or out, approximately halfway between Grants Grove and Cedar Grove. The charming lodge is rustic but beautiful, with flowerbeds mixed in with old, rusted mining equipment. The little cabins were authentic dwellings of early-20th-century miners.

A little farther on is Boyden Cavern. I took the guided tour. American Indians avoided the place, feeling that bad spirits lived there. I can see why. I swallowed hard when the guide turned off the lights and described the mile or so of solid granite over our heads. The

Visit nearby Boyden Cavern for a family-friendly excursion.

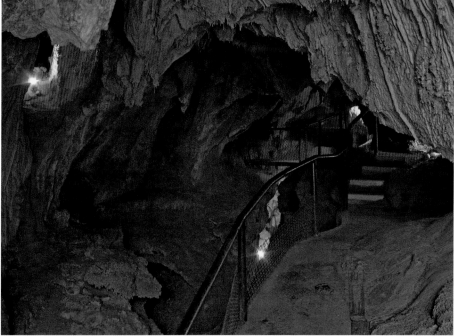

photographed by David Prasad/Flickr/CC BY-SA 2.0 (creativecommons.org/licenses/by-sa/2.0)

KEY INFORMATION

LOCATION: Kings Canyon National Park, about 86 miles east of Fresno on CA 180

CONTACT: 559-565-3341, nps.gov/seki

OPERATED BY: National Park Service

OPEN: Late May–mid November (weather permitting)

SITES: 120

EACH SITE: Picnic table, fire ring, bear box

ASSIGNMENT: First come, first served; no reservations

REGISTRATION: At entrance

FACILITIES: Water, flush toilets, coin-operated showers, wheelchair-accessible sites

PARKING: At site

FEE: $18

ELEVATION: 4,600'

RESTRICTIONS:

PETS: On leash only

FIRES: In fire pits only, may be restricted during high fire danger

ALCOHOL: No restrictions

VEHICLES: 1 per site maximum

OTHER: 6 campers per site maximum; 14-day stay limit

---

children on the tour were thrilled. (A fire in 2015 caused damage to the attraction, and it was still closed at press time, so check to see if it's reopened before heading out.)

Another fun activity for children at Cedar Grove is a horse ride at Cedar Grove Pack Station. Here, you can arrange anything from a 1-hour ride to a weeklong trip into the backcountry. They offer kiddy rides as well. If you come to camp and want to arrange a more elaborate ride, it's best to phone ahead and make reservations. Call 559-565-3464.

Kings River was running too fast for much fishing the last time I was at Cedar Grove, in August. However, the cowboys at the stables told me you could do all right if you knew where to fish. "Where's that?" I asked, but they laughed and wouldn't disclose any information.

Upriver from Moraine, there are several parking areas where you can pull over and walk down to the river. The second or third areas access a part of the river where the current runs languidly even at flood tide. I wonder if this is the cowboy fishing hole? I got my lure wet, but there were no trout takers.

Farther on, past the bridge on the left, you'll find the beginning of the Motor Nature Trail, a dirt road that heads back to Cedar Grove Village across the North Fork Kings River. It passes several great places to park and hang out down by the water.

You can't leave Cedar Grove without hiking up to Mist Falls. The trailhead is at Roads End, about 6 miles from the ranger station in Cedar Grove. Right away, you'll cross Copper Creek, near the site of a former American Indian village. Look carefully and you'll find flakes of obsidian, which American Indians used to make weapons and tools. There was a store here once, and John Muir swore by the pies the owner's wife, Viola, made. About 2 miles in, head uphill following the river. On your left is Buck Peak (8,776'), and the Sphinx (9,146') is behind you. See if you can sort out the ponderosa, Jeffrey, and sugar pines. To the east, don't miss the waterfall on Gardiner Creek. Soon enough, you'll reach Mist Falls, and the sight is worth the climb.

The best time to visit Moraine Campground at Cedar Grove is in the spring. It's cool enough then to hike comfortably all day long, and the crowds haven't begun to arrive in droves, as in August. Still, Kings Canyon National Park is beautiful any month of the year.

Moraine Campground

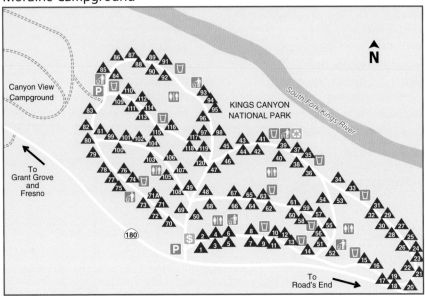

GETTING THERE

From Los Angeles, take I-5 north over the Tejon Pass to CA 99. Drive north past Bakersfield for 104 miles to Fresno. Go east on CA 180 about 85 miles to Cedar Grove Village in Kings Canyon National Park. From Cedar Grove Village continue east on CA 180 for 1 mile to the campground.

GPS COORDINATES: N36° 47' 09" W118° 39' 36"

Kings River runs behind Boyden Cavern and through the campground.

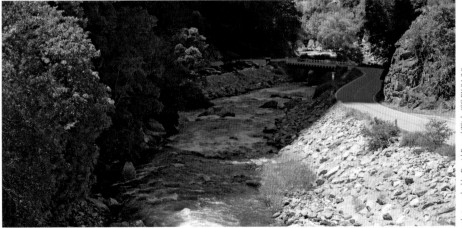

33

Princess Campground

Beauty ★★★★ / Privacy ★★★★ / Spaciousness ★★★★ / Quiet ★★★ / Security ★★★ / Cleanliness ★★★★

This campground has everything—big trees, warm lakes, and fantastic gorge views.

You'll love Princess Campground just like you love a golden retriever for being a basic good dog. Set under the shade of second-growth sequoias and pines, Princess is covered on one flank by a shimmering alpine meadow. The campsites are private and level, and everything is well maintained and clean.

Hume Lake, 3 miles down the road, is a big draw for anybody with an inflatable water toy or a fishing rod. A huge Christian campground occupies one end of the lake's shoreline. Dammed up by lumber folks, Hume Lake supplied the water for the flume that scooted timber down to Sanger in the San Joaquin Valley 54 miles away. Flumes work on the same principle as water slides: water reduces friction.

Unlike the water in the mountain streams, Hume Lake warms up enough that you can actually swim without turning gelid. A path encircles the lake, and you can find your own grassy beach spot. Air mattresses or inexpensive blowup boats are big hits. I saw people catching edible-sized fish as well.

Spacious site 44 has all the amenities: shade, a picnic table, and a fire ring. It's also close to the restrooms and water.

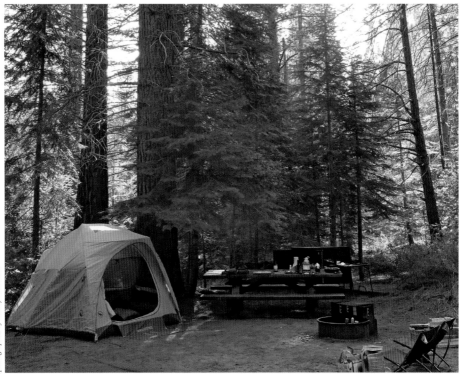

photographed by Kathryn Robinson

KEY INFORMATION

LOCATION: 62 miles east of Fresno on CA 180, Miramonte, CA 93633

CONTACT: 559-784-1500, www.fs.usda.gov/sequoia

OPERATED BY: California Land Management

OPEN: May–October

SITES: 90

EACH SITE: Picnic table, fire ring

ASSIGNMENT: Some sites require reservations; others are first come, first served

REGISTRATION: At entrance or reserve at recreation.gov or 877-444-6777

FACILITIES: Water, vault toilets

PARKING: At site

FEE: $25–$27 plus $9 nonrefundable reservation fee; must pay national park entrance fee

ELEVATION: 5,900'

RESTRICTIONS:

PETS: On leash only

FIRES: In fire pit

ALCOHOL: No restrictions

VEHICLES: RVs up to 32 feet

A choice spot is Sandy Cove Beach. Coming down from CA 180, pass Hume Lake Campground and follow the road around past Powder Canyon Picnic Area, through the Hume Lake Christian Camps, and go along Lakeshore Drive to Sandy Cove Beach. This is a fun and safe place to swim, where the trill of youthful swimmers' voices resounds. Adults seeking more secluded sunbathing can follow Landslide Creek up to find a private spot. The road that heads south to the Generals Highway follows the creek most of the way.

Princess is regarded as an overflow campground for Hume Lake, but I find it offers much better camping. It's quieter and cleaner, and because you have to walk downhill to the lake from Hume Lake Campground, you might as well drive down from Princess. At least up there you won't suffer the incessant camp counselors' whistles in the morning. And the added 700 feet of elevation at Princess cuts down on the bugs and the dust.

The Indian Basin Grove Trail is an easy 1-hour hike, starting about 0.5 mile west of the Princess Campground entrance. You can walk there from Princess or take a car and park in a turnout just west of the road. The trail follows FS 13S50 north through ponderosas and cedars. Look for the sequoia stumps, then for the second-generation sequoias growing back. After a mile or so, pass FS 13S07, which could take you back to Princess Campground, but persevere and follow the road north to a ridge. When the road turns east, find the trail in a patch of manzanita. The trail continues north to a point overlooking Kings Canyon.

Another good hike is to the Boole Tree. Drive west on CA 180 to FS 13S55, then drive 2.7 miles to the trailhead parking lot. Follow the signed trail. It's an easy 2-mile trip in and out. Be sure to see the tree—it's an incredible sight. Why didn't loggers ever cut it down? Nobody knows, but some say Frank Boole, general manager of the Sanger Lumber Company, spared the tree as a tribute to himself.

Just up the road is Grant Grove, with more incredible sequoias. One tree actually antedates Christ by 1,500 years. The short walk out to Panoramic Point is fun, especially at sunset.

At Grant Grove Village you can buy supplies. Many families stay at Princess Campground. The last time I was there, I camped next to a schoolteacher and his herd of children. He was an erudite chap and taught his wee ones some games originating with the Monache and Yokut tribes. Their favorite involved guessing who on the opposing team held a rock beneath an all-concealing blanket.

Bears, though rarely a danger to humans, are abundant around Princess Campground. To avoid a run-in, be careful with your food. As soon as you eat, take the trash to the bins. Conceal your cooler in your car, or better yet, inside one of the campground's steel bear boxes. The bears recognize coolers and know their purpose. Don't leave anything in your tent that has any kind of odor, such as sunscreen, lipstick, skin cream, and so on. Rangers shoot bears when they become repeat food raiders, so be cool and save a bear.

Princess Campground

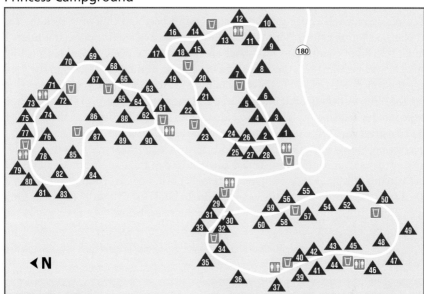

GETTING THERE

From Los Angeles, take I-5 north over the Tejon Pass to CA 99. Drive north past Bakersfield 104 miles to Fresno. Go east on CA 180 for 56 miles to Grant Grove in Kings Canyon National Park. From Grant Grove drive 6 miles north to Princess Campground on the right.

GPS COORDINATES: N36° 18' 13" W118° 56' 29"

34

Quaking Aspen Campground

Beauty ★★★★★ / Privacy ★★★★ / Spaciousness ★★★★ / Quiet ★★★★ / Security ★★★★★ / Cleanliness ★★★★★

Come in the fall for autumn leaves and in the summer for hiking and mountain biking.

Quaking Aspen Campground spans the entire range of camping available in this part of the Sierras. Quaking Aspen is developed, clean, well maintained, and set in a stand of red fir, not quaking aspen as its name infers. Quaking Aspen Campground lies by meadows of willow, aspen, and yarrow.

Brewer's Ponderosa Lodge is a fun place to grab a beer and chili or to pick up ice, but don't plan on shopping there. Springville is the last port of call for supplies. This pretty little town in Tule River country has just about everything you'll need. Before Jedediah Smith trapped beaver here in 1827, the Yaudanchi (a subtribe of the Yokut) lived in the foothills during the winter and trekked to the mountains to gather food in the summer.

By 1857, the settlers poured into the area and, regrettably, occupied the land that once belonged to the Yaudanchis. John Nelson forged his way up the canyon of the Middle Fork of the Tule River (CA 190, east of Springville today) and filed a claim on property that is now Camp Nelson. Springville (named for the soda springs in the area) was the site of a mill that processed the raw timber that was hauled down by horse- and mule-team wagons from the higher reaches of what is today Sequoia National Forest. Logging continued into the early 1900s, when the Porterville Northeastern Railroad built a spur into Springville, allowing lumber, citrus fruits, and apples to be shipped to the valley below.

Quaking Aspen Campground changes from a lush green in spring to a brilliant gold in autumn when the leaves of its signature trees turn.

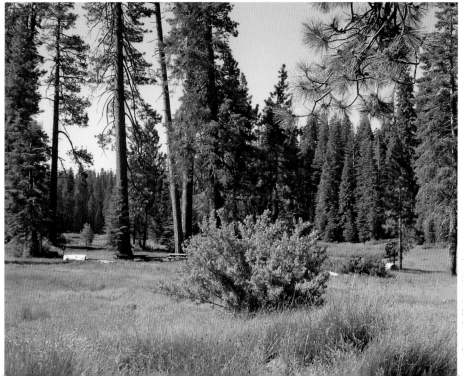

photographed by Jessica Mirmak

KEY INFORMATION

LOCATION: Sequoia National Forest,
27 miles east of Springville on CA 190

CONTACT: 559-784-1500 or 559-539-2607,
www.fs.usda.gov/sequoia

OPERATED BY: U.S. Forest Service

OPEN: April–November

SITES: 32

EACH SITE: Picnic table, fire ring

ASSIGNMENT: Some sites require reservations; others are first come, first served

REGISTRATION: At entrance or reserve at
recreation.gov or 877-444-6777

FACILITIES: Water, vault toilets

PARKING: At site

FEE: $26 plus $9 nonrefundable
reservation fee

ELEVATION: 7,000'

RESTRICTIONS:

PETS: On leash only

FIRES: In fire pits

ALCOHOL: No restrictions

VEHICLES: RVs up to 27 feet

OTHER: 2 wheelchair-accessible sites;
14-day stay limit

Now, citrus orchards dot the lower foothills leading into town along CA 190. Ranching operations spread across wide-open parcels of oak- and buckeye-studded hills. Apples are grown farther up on the cooler, protected slopes, merging into the manzanita, black oak, cedar, and pine. Logging continues under the supervision of the Sequoia National Forest.

Between Quaking Aspen Campground and Brewer's Ponderosa Lodge, note the actual quaking aspens that give the campground its name. These slender trees have light bark and roundish leaves. Vivid green in spring and bright gold in fall, the leaves quiver at the least breath of breeze.

The good bathing holes on Peppermint Creek are downstream from the campground about 0.25 mile. Stick to the south side of the creek, because it's hard to cross over from the other side. The wet rocks are extremely slippery. Don't even think of crossing on them. Find a place with a sandy bottom before you try getting in the water. Also, watch out for the granite slabs on the banks. Their surface decomposes, leaving slippery bits of rock.

A great hike goes out to the Needles Lookout. It's only a 4-mile round-trip of pretty easy walking, but plan on making a day of it. Take lunch. The dirt road to the trailhead heads east about 0.5 mile south of Brewer's Ponderosa Lodge. Drive 2.8 miles in and park. The trail begins at the east end of the parking lot. Note the small purple flowers along the trail. Called pennyroyals (*Mentha pulegium*), they are used to make mint tea. Pennyroyals are not local, however; they are natives of Europe brought in by the forty-niners.

Along the trail, look north to Mount Kaweah and Mount Whitney and northeast to the Kern Plateau peaks of Kern and Olancha. Then, keep an eye out for the lookout on top of the westernmost Needle—it's a fire tower manned in fire season.

Believe me, the view is worth the slog up the switchback ladders to the catwalk. Talk to the firewatcher if he is on duty. This place can get hairy. In storms, the lookout is frequently struck by lightning. In fact, the firewatcher has a special stool fitted with glass insulators that he sits on when lightning is striking nearby!

I enjoyed camping at Quaking Aspen in the summer, but it is especially beautiful in the fall with the turning of the leaves.

Quaking Aspen Campground

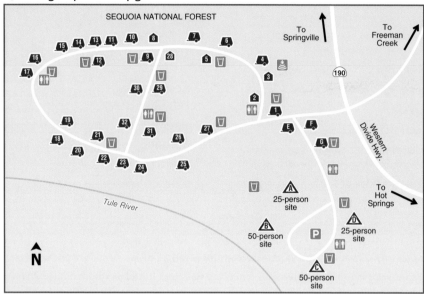

GETTING THERE

From Los Angeles, take I-5 north over the Tejon Pass to CA 99. Drive north on CA 99 past Bakersfield. Take CA 65 north to Porterville. Go east 17 miles on CA 190 to Springville. From Springville, drive 23.3 miles east on CA 190 to Quaking Aspen Campground on the right.

GPS COORDINATES: N36° 07' 17" W118° 32' 46"

Rancheria Campground

Beauty ★★★★ / Privacy ★★★★ / Spaciousness ★★★★ / Quiet ★★★★★ / Security ★★★★ / Cleanliness ★★★★★

Though sometimes crowded, lakeside Rancheria Campground offers solid, safe tent camping.

Rancheria Campground on Huntington Lake is big, handsome, and noisy. The acoustics around camp on the pine-shored lake are such that you can hear a mouse belch at dusk from the south shore. You'll hear folks laughing on boats at the nearby marina, outboards putting on fishing skiffs, and chaps hammering siding on cottages by the town of Lakeshore. It feels like one big beautiful neighborhood.

The campground has been around for a long time, and the sites are screened by pine and brush. Many are walk-ins along the lake, allowing you to pitch your tent right on the shore. Folks with boats can tie them to a root next to their campsite. The beach slopes gently into the water, which makes for good wading. There are sites back in the woods too for people who want to avoid all the aquatic activity.

Rancheria Falls tumbles 150 feet, just east of Huntington Lake.

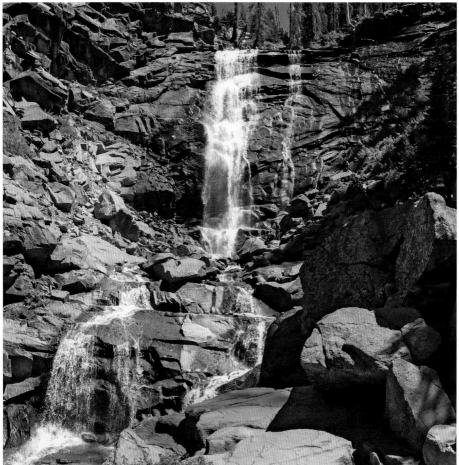

photographed by Sam McMillan (flickr.com/photos/sammcmillanjr)

KEY INFORMATION

LOCATION: 63001 Huntington Lake Road, Lakeshore, CA 93634

CONTACT: 559-297-0706 or 559-893-2111, www.fs.usda.gov/sierra; conditions: 800-427-7623; outside California, 916-445-7623; dot.ca.gov/cgi-bin/roads.cgi

OPERATED BY: California Land Management

OPEN: June–October

SITES: 124 (some tents only)

EACH SITE: Picnic table, fire ring

ASSIGNMENT: Reservations highly recommended

REGISTRATION: At entrance or reserve at recreation.gov or 877-444-6777

FACILITIES: Water, flush and vault toilets

PARKING: At or near site

FEE: $30 plus $9 nonrefundable reservation fee

ELEVATION: 7,000'

RESTRICTIONS:

PETS: On leash only

FIRES: In fire pit

ALCOHOL: No restrictions

VEHICLES: RVs up to 40 feet

OTHER: Camp in color-coded sites—yellow for tents, blue for RVs up to 20 feet, white for RVs up to 30 feet, red for RVs up to 40 feet; 14-day stay limit

Perched on the edge of the wilderness, Huntington Lake is a good first camp for anyone heading farther in to Lake Thomas A. Edison (also known as Edison Lake) or Florence Lake. You'll find last-chance shopping at the Lakeshore Resort General Store and Coffee Shop in Lakeshore and information at the ranger station. There's a good chance that you will want to settle in at Rancheria and forget the hairy drive up over Kaiser Pass.

The lakes in this region comprise the Big Creek Hydroelectric Project, owned and operated by Southern California Edison. Water runs from Lake Edison and Florence Lake before flowing into Huntington Lake and on to Shaver Lake, turning turbines along the way.

C. B. Shaver was the first to use the power of water here when he built a millpond to saw lumber before floating it down a 40-mile flume to Clovis. When the lumber gave out, the power company moved in and built dams and reservoirs.

For a power company, water in a reservoir is like money in the bank. It provides cheap, clean, reliable power that can be used almost immediately. As long as the lakes are full, the vacationing public is happy. But, nothing is worse for power companies and tourism than an empty lake.

You can rent boats at the marina across from Rancheria Campground. Or, visit in the winter and ski at nearby China Peak Mountain Resort. I found the skiing spectacular, but I heard some experts complaining that the best runs were too short. Hike up to Rancheria Falls from the trailhead across the road from Rancheria Campground. Or, hike to the river pools. The trailhead is in the second parking lot of the ski resort.

There is decent shopping at Ken's Market in Shaver Lake, and you'll find drinks, ice, and sundries at the friendly country store in Lakeshore. But, if you want a sirloin steak, you better bring it with you. While you're packing, it's not a bad idea to bring a pair of shoes to wear in and around the lake.

And, don't accommodate the bears! Put all edibles in your car and out of view. Bring a small bottle of bleach and wipe down your cooking gear and picnic table before turning in. Bears don't like the smell.

Be sure to read the memorial on the rock by the ranger station. It honors a crew of airmen who died in 1944. Apparently, a B-24 bomber ran into trouble. The pilot gave the crew two options—bail out or stay with the ship and gut it out. Two men jumped and lived. The plane disappeared into the blue and was lost for a decade. Finally, in 1955, the power company lowered the water in Huntington Lake to make some repairs on the dam. The receding water revealed the wreckage of the missing B-24 and the bodies of the remaining crewmembers.

I thought of those young men as I swam in azure Huntington Lake and stood in the mist from the generator turbines by Kaiser Pass Road. Maybe it would be better if they hadn't been found. Then, we could always think of them out there somewhere, handsome and young in sheepskin flying jackets, their faces full of promise.

Rancheria Campground

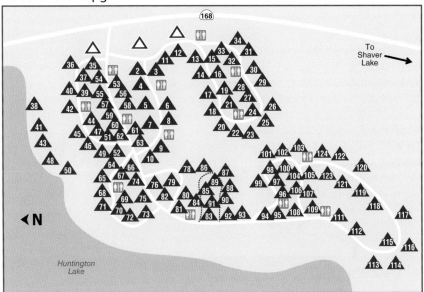

GETTING THERE

From Los Angeles, take I-5 north over the Tejon Pass to CA 99. Drive north past Bakersfield 104 miles to Fresno. Take CA 41 north to CA 168. Go northeast to Shaver Lake and head 20 miles north on CA 168. Rancheria Campground is on the left as you come to the head of Huntington Lake.

GPS COORDINATES: N37° 14' 52" W119° 09' 43"

Redwood Meadow Campground

Beauty ★★★★★ / Privacy ★★★ / Spaciousness ★★★★ / Quiet ★★★★ / Security ★★★ / Cleanliness ★★★★

Visit this happy campground with a meadow full of flowers, near the Trail of 100 Giants.

If campgrounds could have expressions, then Redwood Meadow would have a smiling face. This is an easy campground to like. The facilities are clean and well maintained. The sites are located under well-spaced trees, allowing shadow and sunlight with lots of room for tent pitches. Below is a big meadow with flowers that fills the area with light. All this, and the campground is not that crowded. There are so many free surrounding campgrounds, as well as a lot of dispersed camping, that Redwood Meadow doesn't get hit hard. But for me, it's worth the bucks to stay in this happy campground with the Trail of 100 Giants just across the road.

The Trail of 100 Giants is a great place to get acquainted with the "Big Trees." The largest tree in the grove has a diameter of 20 feet and is 220 feet in height. The trees' ages range between 500 and 1,500 years old. These old guys were seedlings in the early Middle Ages.

Back in the glacial eras, the giant sequoias (*Sequoiadendron gigantuem*) grew all over what is now the Western United States. When the climate dried out, the sequoias retreated to ecological islands with abundant rainfall and runoff, where they grow mostly in granite basins or where bedrock is near the surface.

Try to burn a piece of redwood bark and you'll see how resistant it is to fire. The bark is impregnated with tannins that are resistant to both fire and insects. That allows the trees to grow very old. And, given abundant moisture, redwoods are some of the fastest-growing trees in the United States. Age and growth rate explain why the giant sequoias are so huge.

Take a cue from Baxter the dog and grab a blanket when the sun sets.

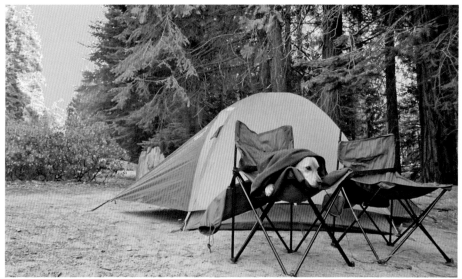

photographed by Alyse Gagne

KEY INFORMATION

LOCATION: About 50 miles east of Springville on Great Western Divide Highway

CONTACT: 559-539-3004 or 559-784-1500, www.fs.usda.gov/sequoia

OPERATED BY: U.S. Forest Service

OPEN: May 15–November 15 (weather permitting)

SITES: 12

EACH SITE: Picnic table, fire ring

ASSIGNMENT: Some sites require reservations; others are first come, first served

REGISTRATION: At entrance or reserve at recreation.gov or 877-444-6777

FACILITIES: Vault toilets, water (phone ahead)

PARKING: At site

FEE: $25–$27 plus $9 nonrefundable reservation fee

ELEVATION: 6,500'

RESTRICTIONS:

PETS: Allowed

FIRES: In fire pits

ALCOHOL: No restrictions

VEHICLES: RVs up to 16 feet

For years, foresters tried to protect the giant sequoia from fire. Fifty years ago, though, they realized that the sequoias need fire to perpetuate. Ground fires do not burn through the bark, but the rising heat opens the cones, which remain on the trees for up to 20 years. When the cones open, the seeds fall on the soft, recently burned earth. When it rains, these seeds germinate in the sunlight that shines to the ground freely through the recently burned foliage.

An interesting friend of the giant sequoia is the giant carpenter ant, who makes nests in the sequoias by hollowing them out. Try not to think about the ant when you're standing under a giant sequoia, and pray for an occasional fire, since it reduces the population of the giant ants.

For bicycling, the Western Divide Highway is a great option. The road is wide, with no blind curves. On a weekday you'll hardly see a car. A good tour is from Redwood Meadow Campground to Brewer's Ponderosa Lodge and back. The round-trip is about 24 miles. You'll bike from good clear water available at the campground to the lodge's varied liquid refreshments and breakfast, lunch, and dinner choices, then back home again to the campground. On the way, a short section of dirt road takes you to Dome Rock—be sure to stop. A quick walk along an obvious path will lead you to a spectacular view. Look down and you'll see the slash of Kern Canyon. Spot the Needles and Peppermint Creek below. What a wild, lovely vista!

Another great mountain-biking trip is down the connector road that heads left from the Western Divide Highway about 3 to 4 miles from Redwood Campground. It climbs Nobe Young Creek basin to Windy Gap, then passes Coy Flat Campground, and ends up at Camp Nelson (about 24 miles one-way). I found the trip to be quite long, and was greatly relieved when someone in our party hitched a ride on a pickup truck back to Redwood Campground to get a relief vehicle.

On big weekends, make sure to reserve a site in advance at Redwood Meadow Campground. I especially like sites 2–8, because they are off the highway and back down to the little stream. If the campground is too busy, head north 0.5 mile on the Western Divide Highway. To the right is a dirt road leading down to Long Meadow Campground, a delightful place to pitch a tent. Or, try Holey Meadow Campground. Or, head back to Parker Pass

Road and go east. Almost immediately, you'll find turnoffs to good dispersed camping on the right by the stream. Armed with a fire permit, you can find great camping spots anytime in this area.

Redwood Meadow Campground

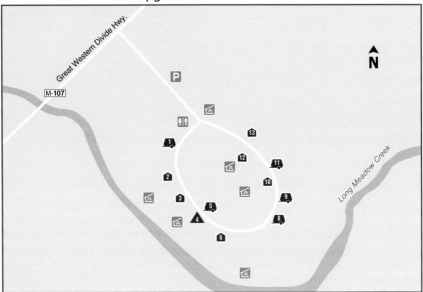

GETTING THERE

From Los Angeles, take I-5 north to CA 99. Drive north past Bakersfield. Take CA 178 east to Lake Isabella. Take CA 155 to Wofford Heights. Bear right to Kernville and drive north on Sierra Way 19.4 miles. Turn left on Parker Pass Road. Drive 10.4 miles to the Great Western Divide Highway. Turn right, and the campground is 3 miles up on the right.

GPS COORDINATES: N35° 58' 36" W118° 35' 32"

37

△ Saddlebag Lake Campground

Beauty ★★★★ / Privacy ★★★ / Spaciousness ★★★★ / Quiet ★★★★★ / Security ★★★★★ / Cleanliness ★★★★★

This campground is perched on a knoll overlooking one of a series of jewel-like alpine lakes.

The Sierra Nevada landscape is a pristine and dramatic mix of glacier-carved granite, snow-fed streams and lakes, wildflower-dotted meadows, and ancient forests; this is one of the most beautiful places in the world. At a high alpine elevation, the campground season is short, just a five-month stretch from June (sometimes later) to mid-October. Camping here is like eating the first local strawberries of spring after a winter of tasteless hothouse fruit: intense, sweet, and fleeting. It may spoil you for anyplace else.

Saddlebag Lake is one of five intimate, nonreserveable Inyo National Forest camp-grounds a mere 2 miles east of the Yosemite National Park entrance station at Tioga Pass. At Tioga Lake, a cluster of open sites sprawls on the lake (but also right off CA 120). Junction Campground, at the intersection of Saddlebag Lake Road and CA 120, is a short distance off both roads, but has more trees to provide privacy. Less than a mile east of Saddlebag Lake Road sits Ellery Lake, slightly downhill from CA 120. This campground has some sites well screened by shrubby willows, directly on Lee Vining Creek. Proceeding 1.6 miles up Saddlebag Lake Road, you'll find the easy-to-miss Sawmill Walk-in Campground, on the left. It's a short, level walk to a gorgeous 12-spot campground with well-spaced sites sprinkled across a rocky alpine meadow dotted with pine. At the end of Saddlebag Lake Road sits the crown jewel of the area, Saddlebag Lake, its namesake campground, and trailheads for the 20-lakes basin.

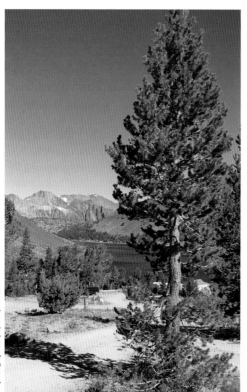

Saddlebag Lake offers respite for campers (and bears!), so store your food properly.

photographed by Fjóla Björnsdóttir

Saddlebag Lake Campground, on a hill above the lake, is reached via a steep gravel road. Although there is plenty of daytime activity down by the lake, the campground is exceptionally quiet. Sites radiate off a single loop, and the ground is somewhat sloped, but gravel tent pads provide level pitches. The premier sites are 16, 18, and 19, which overlook the lake, but most of the other sites offer at least partial views to the water as well as the rugged peaks to the north. Spindly lodgepole pines offer only moderate screening between sites, but heck, everyone's looking at the lake anyway.

The lake is actually a dammed reservoir, its water flowing into Lee Vining Creek and then down to the small town

KEY INFORMATION

LOCATION: Saddlebag Lake Road, Lee Vining, CA 93541

CONTACT: Mono Basin Scenic Area visitor center, 760-873-2538; www.fs.usda.gov/inyo

OPERATED BY: U.S. Forest Service

OPEN: June 1–October 15 (weather permitting); if planning early- or late-season camping, call to be sure the campground is open

SITES: 20 sites for tents or RVs (no designated RV spots, hookups, or dump station)

EACH SITE: Picnic table, fire ring, food-storage locker

ASSIGNMENT: First come, first served; no reservations

REGISTRATION: Self-register at information station

FACILITIES: Drinking water, vault toilets

PARKING: At individual sites

FEE: $22; if arriving from the west, $25–$30 entrance fee for Yosemite

ELEVATION: 10,087'

RESTRICTIONS:

PETS: On leash only during the day and in your tent at night

FIRES: In designated fire rings only

ALCOHOL: No restrictions

OTHER: 14-day stay limit

of Lee Vining, where it generates power for Southern California. A small café squats above Saddlebag Lake's shoreline, providing simple meals three times a day, small boat rentals, and a water taxi service across the lake. From the campground it's a 5-minute walk to the lake for daylong fishing and hiking adventures. Rainbow trout are stocked, but the lake also holds brook, brown, and golden trout.

The elevation here is more than 10,000 feet, and until you adjust, hiking can be a lung-busting experience. A trail departs from the day-use parking lot, heading around the east side of Saddlebag Lake, a less than 4-mile, nearly level hike. The east leg starts out above the lake bisecting a sloping hillside, where you might see Indian paintbrush and yellow wallflower blooming in summer. Small waterfalls gush downhill into the lake, where even from the trail we could see fish swimming in the clear, sapphire-blue water. The trail gradually passes through a pocket of pines, then approaches the far end of the lake. Here you can extend the 4-mile experience to an 8-mile hike past a series of spectacular alpine lakes. The trail can be hard to follow near Helen and Shamrock Lakes, but there is little elevation change to contend with. Back on the west side of Saddlebag Lake, the trail crosses streams and then slips across a talus slope of rocks shed from the mountain on the right. The journey ends near the dam. Continue downhill across the creek to the road, then walk back to the left, and up the campground road (the worst hill of the day). If you are really feeling the elevation or don't care to hike, take the water taxi ($9 round-trip) from the boat launch near the café. The taxi makes exploring the beautiful lakes basin easy.

The café sells firewood but not groceries. If you need ice or other supplies, Lee Vining, 12 miles east along I-395, has a few small stores, restaurants, and gas. Arriving from the west, your best bet for gas and groceries is the central valley town of Oakdale. Once you begin the climb into Yosemite, there are few places to buy food, and gas prices seem to rise with the elevation. Gas is available year-round at Crane Flat and (until early October) Tuolumne Meadows, but you'll pay a premium. You can also eat in the restaurant at the Tioga Pass Resort (on the north side of CA 120, just west of Saddlebag Lake Road), and buy ice and limited other supplies there.

The campground at Saddlebag Lake has food-storage lockers. Use them! At 11:30 p.m. a bear walked past our tent, then overturned a cooler in the adjacent campsite. The big bear was run off, but returned at 4 a.m. and ransacked another campsite. We lay in our tent listening to the mayhem. The camp host advises that air horns are particularly effective aids to chase off marauding bears, but the idea of an air horn blast punctuating the quiet of a campground in the middle of the night is less than appealing. For the sake of your fellow campers (and the local bears), keep your food secured in the bear box.

Saddlebag Lake Campground

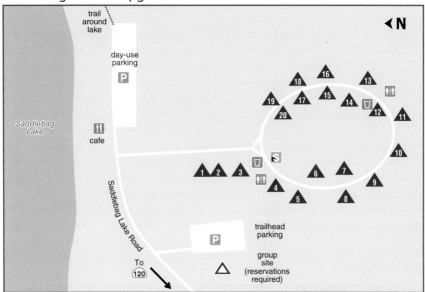

GETTING THERE

From I-5 in San Joaquin County, exit onto CA 120. Drive east through Yosemite. Pass the Tioga Pass entrance station and turn left onto Saddlebag Lake Road. Drive north 2 miles and turn right into the campground. From I-395 in Mono County, turn west on CA 120 and travel 11 miles. Turn right onto Saddlebag Lake Road and drive north 2 miles; turn right into the campground.

GPS COORDINATES: N37° 57' 50" W119° 16' 20"

38

Tillie Creek Campground

Beauty ★★★★★ / Privacy ★★★ / Spaciousness ★★★★ / Quiet ★★★★ / Security ★★★ / Cleanliness ★★★★

Tillie Creek is child-friendly and perfect for all seasons.

I love Tillie in the fall, when the leaves change; in the winter and spring, when it's warm on the plateau and there's snow up above in the mountains that ring the lake; and in the summer, when it's hotter than Hades and all you can do is sit by the water with a beer and a fishing pole.

I also love camping at Tillie Creek with my young niece, because Tillie Creek is ideal for children. There's a beautiful stream running through the camp that's never fast or deep enough to carry off a child. The lake has a gradually sloping shore. The roads through the campground are just right for young cyclists. There are flushing toilets and hot showers.

This is not the forest primeval. Tillie Creek is what a scout camp or small-town park used to be 30 years ago. There are child-friendly activities in the area, and Wofford Heights is just around the corner for a quick ice cream or a fast-food run.

Look out over Isabella Lake and see the watery grave of ancient American Indian villages, historic towns, ranches, and farms—all now submerged. When the dam was built in 1953, water filled the Kern River Valley. When the lake is low, look for a series of snags to find the former courses of the North and South Forks of the Kern.

As you drive toward present-day Kernville, note the old cemetery to the right. Around the cemetery sit the foundations of old Kernville. When Isabella Lake was created, the

In 1924 Tom Walker killed his brother, and the "shootin' Walkers" are now said to haunt this cabin where they once lived.

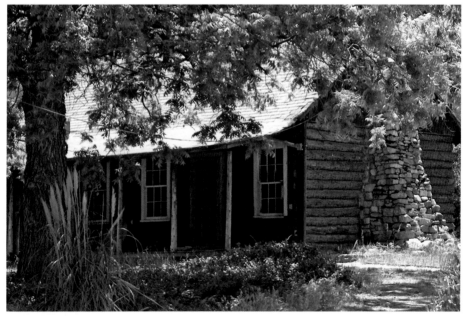

photographed by Melissa Ghergich/Bureau of Land Management/Flickr/CC BY 2.0 (creativecommons.org/licenses/by/2.0)

KEY INFORMATION

LOCATION: Wofford Blvd., Wofford Heights, CA 93285

CONTACT: 559-784-1500, www.fs.usda.gov/sequoia

OPERATED BY: U.S. Forest Service

OPEN: Year-round

SITES: 159

EACH SITE: Picnic table, fire ring

ASSIGNMENT: First come, first served; reservations recommended

REGISTRATION: Host will collect on rounds or reserve at recreation.gov or 877-444-6777

FACILITIES: Water, flush toilets, hot showers, sanitary disposal station, playground, fish-cleaning station, RV dump station

PARKING: At site

FEE: $25–$27 plus $9 nonrefundable reservation fee

ELEVATION: 2,650'

RESTRICTIONS:

PETS: On 6-foot or shorter leash only

FIRES: In fire ring

ALCOHOL: No restrictions

VEHICLES: RVs up to 30 feet

government helped relocate the town to its present site. To get a free map of old Kernville, visit the Kern Valley Museum in Kernville.

In Wofford Heights, head east on Evans Road to visit a site of infamy. Park near the Douglas El Segundo Rod & Gun Club and climb the hill just to the south, called the Hill of Three Crosses. Look for mortars in the rock where the Tübatulabal tribe once ground acorns. Here in 1863, Captain Moses McLaughlin and his men massacred a group of American Indians. At the time, many felt the violence was justified. This can be the basis for a good civics lesson.

To find another historic landmark, drive south on CA 155 to Keyesville Road. Turn right (southwest) and drive to the end of the paved road. Turn right toward Fort Hill to find all that remains of Keyesville. In 1854, Richard Keyes hit gold-bearing quartz a few hundred yards northwest up Hogeye Gulch. To the south, the Mammoth Mine was found soon afterward and the wild town was born. One of the local hunters who supplied the miners with fresh meat was named Grizzly Adams, because he had two pet grizzly bears. (Remember the 1970s TV show about him?) Keyesville is long gone, save one house. Built in 1880, it was the scene of a big gunfight involving the "shootin' Walkers." Today, it is occupied and cared for by some locals.

Another interesting trip is to the South Fork Wildlife Area. Go into Kernville and head south on Sierra Way to the wildlife area around South Fork Kern River. Take field glasses and look for the great blue herons that nest in the crowns of trees. Open-minded herons often share trees with owls or hawks. South of the wildlife area are cottonwood and willow stands managed by the Nature Conservancy. The endangered yellow-billed cuckoo and the southwestern willow flycatcher supposedly nest here—I searched for an hour without luck. Apparently, the cuckoos like to eat hairy caterpillars, and the flycatchers fly so fast they are hard to see.

Marinas in the area rent boats for fun excursions. Remember to bring hats, sunscreen, food, and water. Remember, too, that shallow lakes are more prone to dangerous windblown waves than deep lakes are. That has to do with the relationship between waves and the lake bottom (similarly, ocean waves grow taller as they approach the shallows near land).

How can you be in this area and not go river rafting? The trick is to choose a rafting experience that is compatible with the age and daring of you and your companions. I've been on rafting trips that were and others that turned my hair white. Ask around to find an established rafting company with a solid reputation.

You'll have the most fun, however, just hanging around Tillie Creek Campground. The atmosphere encourages relaxation. The playground attracts and engages children. The changing sun and breeze off the lake combine for an incredible show. Tillie is a place to bring children for a weekend and actually relax.

Tillie Creek Campground

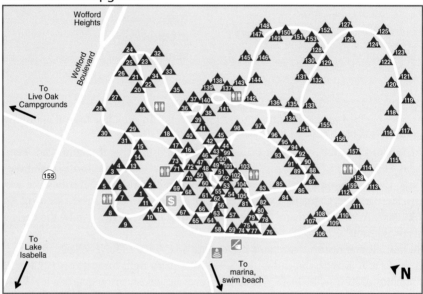

GETTING THERE

From Los Angeles, take I-5 north over the Tejon Pass about 67 miles to CA 99. Drive north on CA 99 about 26 miles to Bakersfield. Take CA 178 about 40 miles east to Lake Isabella. Take CA 155 about 8 miles toward Wofford Heights on the west shore of Isabella Lake. The entrance to Tillie Creek Campground is 1 mile before Wofford Heights on the right.

GPS COORDINATES: N35° 42' 05" W118° 27' 19"

39

⛺ Trapper Springs Campground

Beauty ★★★★★ / Privacy ★★★★★ / Spaciousness ★★★★★ / Quiet ★★★★★ / Security ★★★★★ / Cleanliness ★★★★★

Trapper Springs Campground is an easy-to-access, remote, beautiful campground.

Trapper Springs Campground is clean, uncrowded, and beautiful at a subalpine 8,200 feet. It's a land of granite peaks towering thousands of feet above thick pines, of twisted tamarack and juniper growing out of rock. Courtright Reservoir is a sparkling blue gem against the gray granite, brown tree trunks, and green pine boughs.

What an incredibly beautiful place! John Muir, Scottish-American sheepherder turned naturalist, wrote:

> *The Sierra should be called not the Nevada or Snowy Range, but the range of light. And after ten years spent in the heart of it, rejoicing and wondering, bathing in the glorious floods of light, seeing the sunbursts of morning among the icy peaks, the noonday radiance on the trees and rocks and snow, the flush of the alpenglow, and a thousand dashing waterfalls with their marvelous abundance of irised spray, it still seems to me above all others the Range of Light, the most divinely beautiful of all the mountain chains I have ever seen.*

Rock climbers flock to Trapper Dome.

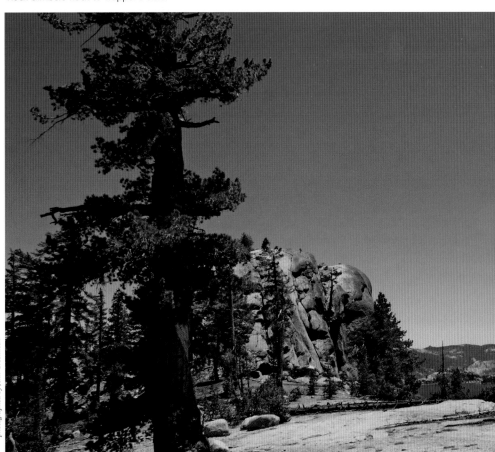

photographed by John Greenheck

KEY INFORMATION

LOCATION: Courtright Way,
Shaver Lake, CA 93664

CONTACT: 916-386-5164,
www.fs.usda.gov/sierra

OPERATED BY: Pacific Gas and Electric

OPEN: May–October

SITES: 70

EACH SITE: Picnic table, fire ring

ASSIGNMENT: First come, first served;
no reservations

REGISTRATION: At entrance

FACILITIES: Water, vault toilets

PARKING: At site; $5 for additional vehicles

FEE: $24

ELEVATION: 8,300'

RESTRICTIONS:

PETS: On leash only; $1 per night

FIRES: In fire pit

ALCOHOL: No restrictions

VEHICLES: RVs up to 22 feet

OTHER: This is bear country—store food
properly; 14-day stay limit

Range of Light. That thought stayed with me for the two days my wife and I spent at Trapper Springs. On the first, we walked down the trail to Courtright Reservoir, hiked across the pined granite escarpments at dusk, and drank sundowners on a rock scoured clean by ice, sun, and wind.

The next day, September 15, hunting season began. I expected campgrounds full of gun-toting, beer-swigging NRAers and fusillades of rifle fire at dawn. Au contraire—the Trapper Springs Campground attracted just a few polite gentlemen hunters, and there were a few far-off rifle pops, but otherwise nothing disturbed the sylvan peace of the reservoir and mountainside.

I'm not sure if this state of serenity had anything to do with Marv, our camp host, and his dog, but it's a possibility. The first night, the campground hostess came by in her golf cart, and we asked her about the hunters. She said, "Well, if they get rowdy, I send my husband Marv down to talk to them, and he takes his dog." Well, we met Marv. He looked rawhide tough, like an ex–rodeo rider, and his dog made your average pit bull look like a French poodle.

The campground was built and is run by Pacific Gas and Electric. They do a fine job. All the facilities are well maintained. The sites are all secluded and clean, and the pitches are well off the service road. The pit toilets are clean. We paid for two sites—9 and 10—sheltered under a huge granite tor.

The campground is located well off the reservoir shore, which keeps the place relatively uncrowded. In Southern California, wherever there's water, there are people. They come for fishing, boating, swimming, and the beauty and primitive peace of mind that a stream or lake provides. So, pick a campground like Trapper Springs that's a little off the water and you won't have too many neighbors.

The trail to the reservoir leaves from the bottom of the second campground loop. The shore is about 0.25 mile downhill. Or, you can just head north up across the granite escarpments and work your way down. A fishing trail encircles the entire reservoir. There are great places to picnic, sunbathe, and fish. If you fish, be sure to obtain a license and to wear it visibly.

Considering how remote Trapper Springs Campground feels, the road in is pretty mild. Dinkey Creek Road is wide and well graded; you'll thank God for this when you meet the heavily loaded lumber trucks. You'll pass the ranger station and small grocery store at Dinkey and head east on McKinley Grove Road. Past the turnoff to Courtright Reservoir Road is the small Wishon Village store and private campground, where you can buy last-minute supplies, including campfire wood. The sign on the door of their saloon reads, "Monday Night Football—Bring your own finger food." Then, head up the hill to Courtright Reservoir; the ascent is gradual, beautiful, and well graded. Before you know it, you're there.

Trapper Springs Campground

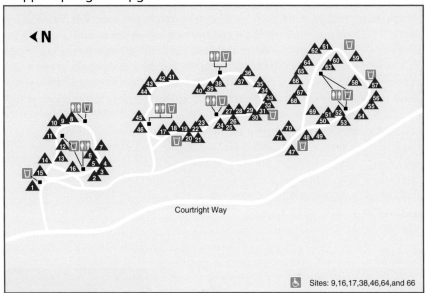

Sites: 9,16,17,38,46,64,and 66

GETTING THERE

From Los Angeles, take I-5 north over the Tejon Pass to CA 99. Drive north on CA 99 past Bakersfield 104 miles to Fresno. Take CA 41 north to CA 168 and go northeast to Shaver Lake. From the town of Shaver Lake, turn east on Dinkey Creek Road and drive 12 miles to McKinley Grove Road. Drive 14 miles to Courtright Way. Go left and proceed 12 miles up Courtright Way to Trapper Springs Campground.

GPS COORDINATES: N37° 06' 01" W118° 59' 05"

40

⛺ Trumbull Lake Campground

Beauty ★★★★★ / Privacy ★★ / Spaciousness ★★★ / Quiet ★★★★★ / Security ★★★★★ / Cleanliness ★★★★

Come here for the lakes, the mountains, and the big sky.

Located by three tiny jade lakes on the backside of Yosemite, Trumbull Lake Campground is popular. It is primitive (no showers), but most of the campsites are reservable. People come back every year. The store in the nearby Virginia Lakes Resort sells basic supplies. The access road is paved and straight. The fishing is good, the hiking superb. Views of the snowy mountains rising around the three lakes take your breath away. Everybody you meet is complicit, because they are in on the secret that this is the most beautiful spot on Earth.

The campground is on a slope above Trumbull Lake. The tiny lake by the Virginia Lakes Resort is over the hill, and the third lake is just a few hundred yards up the gravel road. The campground is like a scruffy dog. You don't like the way it looks, but after a while you learn to love it. The sites are not well engineered. Many are set too close together or too close to the pit toilets—especially the sites down by the lake. You get the feeling the campground evolved haphazardly, but hey, here you are, on the far side of nowhere, pretty close to God.

The drive in is spectacular. Come from Los Angeles, and drive up US 395 through the Mojave Desert, the Owens Valley, and up past Mammoth and Mono Lakes. This is the most spectacularly diverse terrain in California, with tons of stuff to do on the way. You can also head up from Los Angeles along the west side of the Sierras, and come across on CA 120 through Yosemite National Park.

Above 10,000 feet, the Sierras are breathtaking in more ways than one.

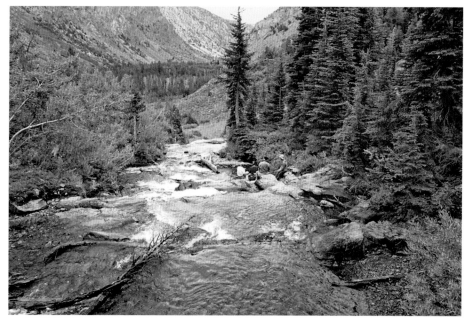

photographed by Charles Patterson

KEY INFORMATION

LOCATION: Virginia Lakes Road, Bridgeport, CA 93517

CONTACT: 775-331-6444, www.fs.usda.gov/htnf

OPERATED BY: U.S. Forest Service

OPEN: Mid-June–mid-October (weather permitting)

SITES: 43

EACH SITE: Picnic table, fire ring

ASSIGNMENT: Some sites offer reservations; others are first come, first served

REGISTRATION: At entrance or reserve at recreation.gov or 877-444-6777

FACILITIES: Water, vault toilets

PARKING: At individual sites, $6 per night for additional vehicle

FEE: $23 plus $9 nonrefundable reservation fee

ELEVATION: 9,500'

RESTRICTIONS:

PETS: On leash only

FIRES: In fire ring

ALCOHOL: No restrictions

VEHICLES: RVs up to 35 feet

OTHER: Don't leave food out; no swimming in lake

From San Francisco, take CA 108 over the Sonora Pass, where the granite meets the clouds at 9,626 feet. This was the Old Sonora-Mono Toll Road, and the men who cut the road had sangfroid. Make sure your flivver is in good shape, and hang on to the steering wheel. It is wild and beautiful—*For Whom the Bell Tolls,* starring Gary Cooper, was filmed here.

I bought salmon eggs and power bait in Lee Vining and caught a decent-sized trout on hooks trimmed of the barb so that I could release (since Tuesday is always spaghetti night). My older sister came along—her first time in the Sierra Nevada in 40 years—and we sat out in the meadow among the lupine and forget-me-nots with a star map and looked up at the sky.

The next day we hiked up to the trailhead by Blue Lake and then hiked a mile up to Frog Lakes. This is up around 10,000 feet, so expect to suck some air. Take your time and rest often. Then we plugged on to Summit Lake on the Sierra Ridge between Camiaca Peak and Excelsior Mountain to the south. We stopped for sandwiches and soda chilled in the cold lake water, and watched storm clouds close in around Excelsior Mountain (elevation 12,446'). We scooted back down to the campground just ahead of a completely unseasonable (early July) thundershower, replete with ear-cracking thunder, hearty gusts of wind, and frightening, white streaks of lightning.

Cringing in our tent under the pines, I regaled my sister with tales of old John Muir, who loved storms and climbed to the top of the highest pine and tied himself in while the elements raged around him, and shouted Whitmanesque exaltations to the primal gods. And John didn't come back to his tent and a towel; he camped in an old overcoat with his sundries in the pockets. He survived one bone-numbing night by crawling into a hot mud spring—alternating cooking one side of himself and freezing the other.

The next morning the sky was as clear blue as the sea, and the chirping sparrows flitted from bush to flower in the meadow. We borrowed an inflatable boat from a camping neighbor and floated around the lake, trailing a little bait and staring up at the mountains above the basin.

I spoke to the campground host (from L & L Inc.), who told me they had plans to make more of the campsites reservable. I checked out all the sites. Sites 10–13 are lakeside with a great view, but there's heavy traffic and they're near a pit toilet. I preferred the campsites off the lake, around the fringes of the camp. Site 4 was my favorite. After that came sites 5, 7, 8 (not site 6), and 35–37. Still, the campsite itself doesn't really matter. Shortly after arriving at Trumbull Lake Campground, as soon as you take a good look around at the mountains and water, you'll know you're home.

Trumbull Lake Campground

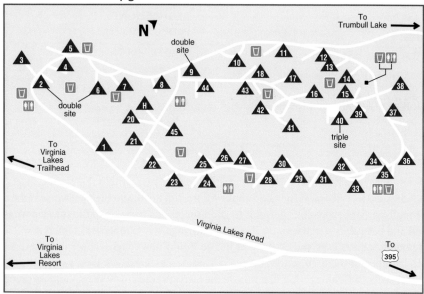

GETTING THERE

From Bridgeport, go 14 miles south on US 395 to the Conway Summit. Turn right onto Virginia Lakes Road and drive 6 miles to the campground on the right. From Lee Vining, drive 12 miles north on US 395 to the Conway Summit and go left on Virginia Lakes Road. Drive 6 miles to the campground on the right.

GPS COORDINATES: N38° 03' 02" W119° 15' 28"

41

Twin Lakes Campground

Beauty ★★★★★ / Privacy ★★★★ / Spaciousness ★★★★★ / Quiet ★★★ / Security ★★★★★ / Cleanliness ★★★★★

Here is a perfect place to spend summer vacation with the family.

The Twin Lakes around Twin Lakes Campground look like blue beans joined at the hip. A little bridge connects the two lakes, and folks in rental rowboats and canoes scoot underneath it. Grandfathers teach their grandchildren how to fish as a waterfall cascades down the cliff above the lakes.

The campground is both accessible and friendly. There are rustic cabins, a lodge, and a store. A few miles away, in the city of Mammoth Lakes, you'll find pizzerias, hardware stores, and a big wonderful Vons Grocery Store on Old Mammoth Road. Twin Lakes Campground is a great place to camp for a week; bring your family for the summer vacation.

The campsites sprawl around the two lakes and uphill across the road. If Twin Lakes Campground is full, head a few hundred yards up the road to beautiful Coldwater Campground on Coldwater Creek. Or head a mile or so up to Lake Mary Campground and Lake George Campground. All the sites are wonderful.

Head to the top of Coldwater Campground and walk a few hundred yards to the old Mammoth Consolidated Gold Mine on Mineral Hill. Here, you can see some of the old buildings from the mining towns and locations of the many bawdy houses and a saloon

This footbridge divides the two Twin Lakes, which look just as beautiful when frozen in winter.

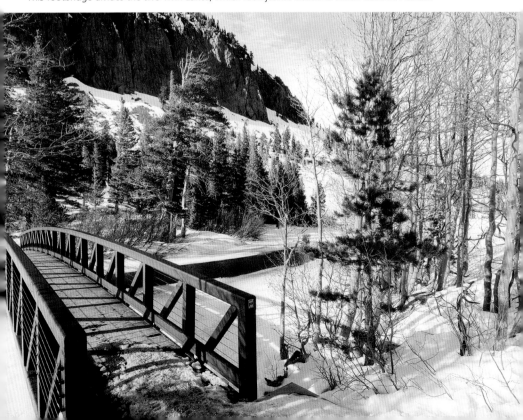

KEY INFORMATION

LOCATION: 518 Twin Lakes Road, Mammoth Lakes, CA 93546

CONTACT: 760-924-5500, www.fs.usda.gov/inyo

OPERATED BY: U.S. Forest Service

OPEN: May 25–October 31

SITES: 94

EACH SITE: Picnic table, fire ring, bear box

ASSIGNMENT: First come, first served or by reservation

REGISTRATION: At entrance or reserve at recreation.gov or 877-444-6777

FACILITIES: Water, flush toilets, boat rental, wheelchair-accessible sites

PARKING: At site

FEE: $24 plus $9 nonrefundable reservation fee

ELEVATION: 8,700'

RESTRICTIONS:

PETS: On leash only

FIRES: In fire pits

ALCOHOL: No restrictions

VEHICLES: RVs up to 22 feet

OTHER: To reduce vehicle traffic into Devils Postpile, a shuttle bus system has been implemented. Campers pay a one-time exception fee of $10 per vehicle. Stop at the Mammoth Lakes visitor center (on the way into Mammoth Lakes) or the Adventure Center (at the ski area) for more information.

named the Temple of Folly (long-since destroyed). Walk around the old buildings and rusted machinery and imagine the men who sweated in the summer sun and froze in the winter, obsessed with gold. Climb to the upper adit in the early morning for a view of Mount Banner and Mount Ritter.

Take the nice little hike to Emerald Lake. It's about a mile up the mountain. The trailhead and parking lot are next to the parking lot for the mine on Mineral Hill. Walk up by Coldwater Creek, where there are lupine, monkeyflower, and fireweed. Bring a picnic and climb the rocks around the lake. Bring fishing gear as well. I watched one woman reel in two decent trout while I ate my sandwich.

Rent a canoe to explore the Twin Lakes and perhaps catch a few fish.

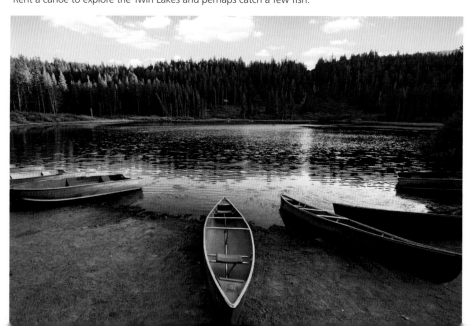

If you are ambitious, go around the left side of Emerald Lake. At the signed junction, go right to Gentian Meadow and Sky Meadows. Climb up by the inlet creek and reach tiny Gentian Meadow. Carry on up past a waterfall, and after a while you'll reach Sky Meadows. Look for paintbrush, corn lily, and elephant's heads among the grass. It's about 2.5 miles back down the hill.

Or if you are truly ambitious, pick up the trail to Duck Pass (8.2 miles round-trip) back in the parking lot by the trailhead to Emerald Lake. Find the Duck Pass sign and start climbing. When you reach the entry sign for the John Muir Wilderness, bear right. Climb through lodgepoles, pines, and hemlocks, and carry on past the trail to Arrowhead Lake, Skelton Lake, and Barney Lake. Next, you'll see alpine Duck Pass ahead, with all the high-elevation flowers—columbine, gentian, and sorrel. Finally, traverse the pass and you'll see Duck Lake and pretty little Pika Lake on the left.

Back at Twin Lakes Campground, you can take a nice stroll around the shore to the falls. Access the trail behind campsite 24. You'll see a sign that says PRIVATE ROAD. Bear left and follow the trail that heads through the trees to the waterfall. Or walk over to Tamarack Lodge. This graceful establishment was built in 1923. The clerk from the grocery store averred that Tamarack Lodge has the best food in Mammoth Lakes.

Twin Lakes Campground

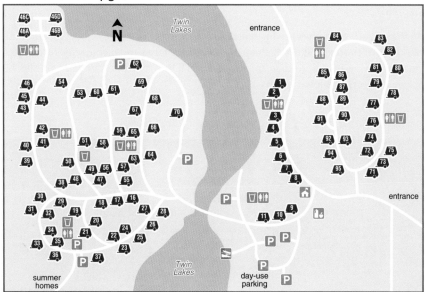

GETTING THERE

From Los Angeles, take I-5 north to CA 14. Go north on CA 14 about 116 miles to US 395 near Inyokern. Go north on US 395 for 123 miles to Bishop. Continue 37 miles north on US 395 to Mammoth Lakes. From Mammoth Lakes, go west 3 miles on Lake Mary Road to the campground.

GPS COORDINATES: N38° 09' 10" W119° 20' 58"

42

⚠ Vermillion Campground

Beauty ★★★★★ / Privacy ★★★★★ / Spaciousness ★★★★ / Quiet ★★★★ / Security ★★★★★ / Cleanliness ★★★★★

Vermillion Campground proves that the best and most beautiful camping is usually the least accessible.

Vermillion Campground is superb tent camping and worth every bit of the terrifying-but-beautiful drive in over Kaiser Pass. Plan on at least a 1.5-hour drive from Huntington Lake. Bring all provisions—only ice and a few sundries are available at Vermilion Valley Resort. Expect your automobile engine to hiccup a bit while climbing the 8,800-foot Kaiser Pass. (Buy premium gasoline for the climb; your car will thank you.) Turn on your lights, since the road is narrow, and remember, cars coming up have the right of way.

When you crest Kaiser Pass on the way to Vermillion, look out over the San Joaquin River Canyon and the Kaiser Wilderness. John Muir wrote:

Westward, the general flank of the range is seen flowing sublimely away from the sharp summits, in smooth undulations; a sea of huge gray granite waves dotted with lakes and meadows, and fluted with stupendous canyons that grow steadily deeper as they recede into the distance.

At Vermillion, most sites are for tents only. This is no easy access for RVs, and most of the parking places are too short or steep for RVs. The pitches and picnic tables are a respectable distance away as well. At the campground you'll find sandy beaches and granite, pined points creating private coves and bays.

Ponderosa pines shelter most of the campsites surrounding Lake Edison.

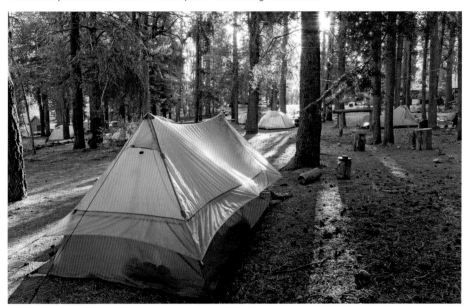

KEY INFORMATION

LOCATION: Edison Lake Road, Prather, CA 93651

CONTACT: 559-297-0706, www.fs.usda.gov/sierra

OPERATED BY: Sierra National Forest

OPEN: June–September

SITES: 31

EACH SITE: Picnic table, fire ring

ASSIGNMENT: First come, first served; reservations recommended

REGISTRATION: At entrance or reserve at recreation.gov or 877-444-6777

FACILITIES: Water, vault toilets

PARKING: At or near site

FEE: $26–$28 plus $9 nonrefundable reservation fee

ELEVATION: 7,000'

RESTRICTIONS:

PETS: On leash only

FIRES: In fire pit

ALCOHOL: No restrictions

VEHICLES: RVs up to 16 feet

OTHER: 15-mph limit for boats on Lake Edison; 14-day stay limit

---

The swimming in Lake Edison was great. Granted, I was there in September, but you don't have to be a polar bear to enjoy jumping in and splashing around. Bring little rubber shoes for the children, so they can race through the shallows.

A friendly couple camping near my wife and me invited us to use their kayaks. We paddled east for about 0.5 mile and beached on an island about 300 yards offshore. I swam and then lay on hot granite slabs and looked across at the snowfields on the mountains ringing the canyon. On a boat trolling by, I saw a guy pull in at least a 3-pound trout. What an incredible place!

The Vermilion Valley Resort runs a water ferry, which leaves the resort at 9:30 a.m. It drops you off to the east at the head of the lake, where the fishing is spectacular. Some folks hike up the trail toward Mono Pass, and some just lie around and wait for the ferry to come pick them up at 4 p.m. The round-trip costs $15, and you can bring your dog for free.

You can also hike east of the campground about a mile to a respectable brook. There is a bridge about 300 yards north, or you can wade across and freeze your feet off. This water comes off a glacier for sure. A little farther, the trail splits. The left fork heads up Silver Pass to the John Muir Trail/Pacific Crest Trail. The right fork takes you 15 miles up to Mono Pass and down the other side to Rock Creek below Mammoth (using the ferry cuts miles off this hike).

The resort rents boats for about $50 a day. This is reasonable, especially when you consider the alternative of trailering a boat up over Kaiser Pass. The resort also has a little café and rents some basic rooms. You can take a classy hot-spring soak in a deep tub at Mono Hot Springs.

Try to pick a campsite at Vermillion well away from the resort, since they run a generator until about 10 p.m. Wood is at a premium, and bundles are expensive at the resort store. Instead, bring a saw. East of the camp, along the trail to the brook, there are quite a few deadfalls. The sand around the pitches is fine and invasive. It's a good idea to bring along a bucket to dip your feet in before entering your tent. Bring a small brush to clean out the tent floor.

Be sure to check with rangers about the water before you arrive. The water at Vermillion is wonderful and spills out of a 400-foot artesian well, but the day we left, an inspector came through and posted the water spigots with NOT SAFE TO DRINK signs. I wished I'd brought a filter to purify the lake water, because the only other alternative was boiling it. Luckily, an hour later, the water scare turned out to be a false alarm.

If Vermillion is full, head back down the road a few miles to Mono Creek Campground. Or, try Mono Hot Springs, which has 26 sites. Because there is no dispersed camping in the area, the only other alternative is Jackass Meadow below the Florence Lake Dam.

Vermillion Campground

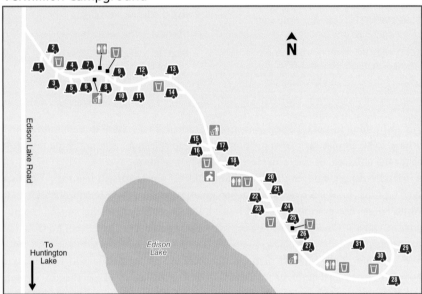

GETTING THERE

From Los Angeles, take I-5 north over the Tejon Pass to CA 99. Drive north on CA 99 past Bakersfield 104 miles to Fresno. Take CA 41 north to CA 168. Go northeast (right) to Shaver Lake. From Shaver Lake, head 20 miles north on CA 168 to Huntington Lake. From Lakeshore on Huntington Lake, take Kaiser Pass Road (FS 80) to Edison Lake Road at Mono Hot Springs. Continue 5 miles north to Vermillion Campground.

GPS COORDINATES: N37° 22' 44" W119° 00' 38"

43

White Wolf Campground

Beauty ★★★★★ / Privacy ★★★★★ / Spaciousness ★★★★★ / Quiet ★★★★★ / Security ★★★★★ / Cleanliness ★★★★★

White Wolf Campground is the only campground in Yosemite National Park worth squeezing into.

Yosemite National Park is heaven on earth. With the Mariposa Battalion, the first English-speaking party to see Yosemite Valley, was Lafayette Bunnell. In 1892, he wrote:

> *The grandeur of the scene was softened by the haze that hung over the valley—light as gossamer—and by the clouds which partially dimmed the higher cliffs and mountains. This obscurity of vision merely increased the awe with which I beheld it, and as I looked, a peculiar exalted sensation seemed to fill my whole being, and I found my eyes in tears with emotion.*

The Yosemite tribe, the original inhabitants, loved the valley too, but the arrival of the forty-niners ended their resiliency. By 1852, Chief Tenaya of the Yosemites, his tribe decimated, was stoned to death by some raiding Mono tribe members. Soon after, Augustus T. Dowd, a miner hunting in the valley, saw a tree bigger than he'd ever seen before. He told his friends about it, and the tourists began flooding in. Yosemite Valley became a mecca to the world.

Wildflowers flourish in the wet meadows and riverbanks surrounding White Wolf Campground. Don't forget the bug spray!

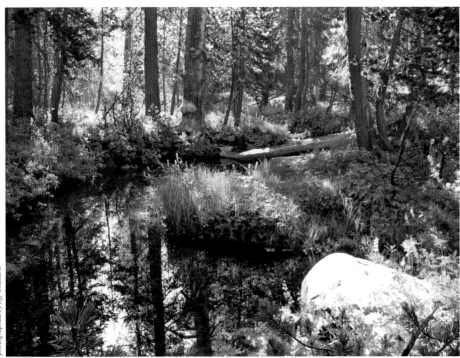

photographed by Jeff Goddard

KEY INFORMATION

LOCATION: White Wolf Road,
Yosemite Valley, CA 95389

CONTACT: 209-372-8502, nps.gov/yose; for
recorded information, call 209-372-0200

OPERATED BY: National Park Service

OPEN: July–September

SITES: 74

EACH SITE: Picnic table, fire ring,
food-storage locker

ASSIGNMENT: First come, first served;
no reservations

REGISTRATION: At entrance

FACILITIES: Water, flush toilets

PARKING: At site

FEE: $18 plus $25–$30 Yosemite National Park
entrance fee

ELEVATION: 8,000'

RESTRICTIONS:

PETS: On leash only

FIRES: In fire pit

ALCOHOL: No restrictions

VEHICLES: RVs up to 27 feet

OTHER: 14-day stay limit; store food
properly from bears

Now, 4-hour traffic jams in Yosemite Valley are common, and the campgrounds are constantly booked. Avoid Yosemite Valley, and explore the rest of the park instead. Come in from the east over the Tioga Pass off US 395 or from the west on CA 120. Shun CA 41, and don't get stuck in the Wawona Tunnel.

However, you should see Tuolumne Meadows and camp in White Wolf Campground. John Muir eloquently described the Tioga Pass area:

From garden to garden, ridge to ridge, I drifted enchanted, now on my knees gazing into the face of a daisy, now climbing again and again among the purple and azure flowers of the hemlocks, now down into the treasuries of the snow, or gazing afar over domes and peaks, lakes and woods, and the billowy glaciated fields of the upper Tuolumne, and trying to sketch them. In the midst of such beauty, pierced with its rays, one's body is all one tingling palate. Who wouldn't be a mountaineer! Up here all the world's prizes seem nothing.

White Wolf Campground is full of tiny meadows and stands of lodgepole pine, and the Middle Tuolumne River flows through the campground. The sites are set among the pines and granite boulders. The campground is constructed beautifully; each loop seems miles away from the others. The arrangement of the tables and sites create a sense of spaciousness. The facilities are clean and well tended. This is slow, elegant camping.

Only the little bear wandering around camp caused a little nervousness. Obviously he was a special bear because he had little colored tags in his ears. Our neighbor shook a towel at the little bear, and he decamped, at least for that day. Of course, we were careful to put away our coolers, even if we were only leaving camp for a moment. Bears get a record for raiding campers, and the rangers are forced to take steps. We didn't want that to happen to the little bear with tags in his ears.

We hiked up to Hardin Lake and sat under the pines reading John Muir. Muir cavorted through these mountains, wearing a great coat, and carried all his gear in his pockets. At night, he lay down in the same massive coat and slept. Those old-timers were real men!

Take John A. "Snowshoe" Thompson, for example. Every winter from 1856 to 1876, Thompson carried the U.S. mail alone across the Sierra. Traveling on skis (called snowshoes in those days), Thompson carried a 100-pound pack and made the 180-mile round-trip in five days. His diet consisted of beef jerky and crackers, and he drank snow. He didn't carry a blanket or wear an overcoat.

At night, Thompson would find a tree stump. After setting fire to the stump, he'd cut some fir boughs for a bed. With his feet to the fire, he'd sleep through the worst blizzards. If he was caught outside camp in a bad blizzard, he just stood on a rock and danced a jig to stay warm.

Today, camping life is a little easier. Still, remember to get supplies in the western flatlands or in Mammoth Lakes on your way in from the east. Only limited grocery items are available in Tuolumne Meadows, Crane Flat, and White Wolf Lodge near White Wolf Campground (in the summer months only).

White Wolf Campground

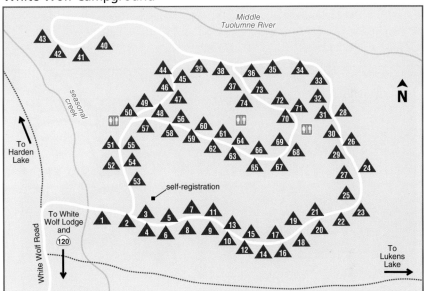

GETTING THERE

From Los Angeles, take I-5 north to CA 14. Go north on CA 14 about 116 miles to US 395 near Inyokern. Go north on US 395 for 123 miles to Bishop. Continue north on US 395 for 57 miles to CA 120 (Tioga Pass Road). Go west 43 miles to White Wolf Road on the right. The White Wolf Campground is about a mile down that road.

GPS COORDINATES: N37° 52' 15" W119° 38' 50"

THE SOUTHERN SIERRAS

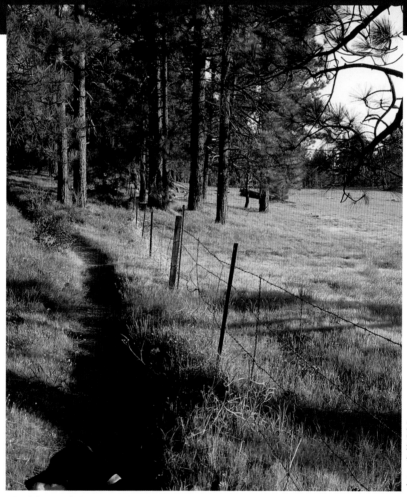

photographed by Bob Perry

This hiking trail skirts the edge of Laguna Meadow (see page 152).

44

Dark Canyon Campground

Beauty ★★★★★ / Privacy ★★★★ / Spaciousness ★★★★ / Quiet ★★★★★ / Security ★★★★★ / Cleanliness ★★★★★

Dark Canyon Campground is a heartbreaker—so beautiful and so near Los Angeles.

I drove through Idyllwild in a mist so thick the neon lights of the cute little mountain town could only blush through the fog. I found a place to park and drifted along a sidewalk until I ran right into a Mount San Jacinto State Park ranger who said this fog never happens this time of year. It was June 15; it was supposed to be sunny and at least 80°F.

Back on CA 243, I leaned out the window and navigated by the stripes down the middle of the highway until FS 4S02 split off to the right, and I could reckon the road by aiming for the gap in the pines. After traveling down the narrowing road and across a stream, I was at Dark Canyon Campground, one of the most charming campgrounds in the very charming Idyllwild area of the San Bernardinos.

Upon arrival, it didn't take long to find the perfect campsite down by the stream that runs through the canyon. The water is cold and runs clear around granite boulders through pools with clean sand bottoms. In this area, and most parts of the San Bernardino National Forest, water is at a premium.

The 17 campsites in Dark Canyon are perfect for tent camping. The fire pits and picnic tables for some of the sites are a 15-yard walk away from the parking lot (ample enough for

From Dark Canyon Campground, head east to explore Mount San Jacinto State Park.

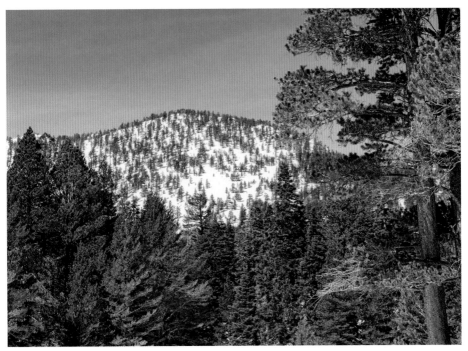

KEY INFORMATION

LOCATION: FS 4S02, Banning, CA 92220

CONTACT: 909-382-2921,
www.fs.usda.gov/sbnf

OPERATED BY: U.S. Forest Service

OPEN: May–mid-October

SITES: 17

EACH SITE: Picnic table, fire ring

ASSIGNMENT: Some sites offer reservations;
others are first come, first served

REGISTRATION: At entrance or reserve at
recreation.gov or 877-444-6777

FACILITIES: Water, vault toilets

PARKING: Within 20 yards of sites

FEE: $12; $5 extra-vehicle fee

ELEVATION: 5,800'

RESTRICTIONS:

PETS: On leash only

FIRES: In fire pit

ALCOHOL: No restrictions

VEHICLES: RVs up to 22 feet

OTHER: Road in is very narrow;
maximum 8 people per site

an RV, however). Five sites are located down by the stream and the rest are up in the pines above the campground.

Shortly after I arrived, it started snowing, and my hike around the canyon was screened through the hard-driving sleet and wet snow. What I saw were pines; Dark Canyon is right on the line between north-facing upper chaparral and the higher yellow pine forest. Both of these areas are packed with pines: Coulter pine, white fir, incense cedar, sugar, and yellow pine. Down by the stream, you'll see riparian trees like alder, willow, and black cottonwood.

I hiked a mile or so up the dirt road to the trailhead that heads east into Mount San Jacinto State Park to Deer Spring. By this time, it was sleeting harder, so I endeavored to collect some dry wood and light a fire in my fire pit. Fortunately, I had a can of charcoal lighter fluid, which, when combined with a little dry paper and a modest amount of kindling, will start up just about any campground wood. I know lighter fluid doesn't sound kosher to the former Boy Scout planning a camping trip at home in the living room, but when everyone is blowing and fanning wet pine needles and wet wood, this petroleum distillate cheater can make you look like a hero. On the other hand, hardware stores also sell a small hatchet-sized splitter, which does a good job chopping wood into more easily lit kindling if you can't handle the humiliation of the tenderfoot charcoal fluid.

Dark Canyon is very popular. The campground hostess told me it usually fills up early Friday afternoon for the weekends. On big weekends, she recommended arriving on Thursday. It's a great idea to make a reservation.

If you decide not to reserve, look for the sign on FS 4S02 informing you if Dark Canyon Campground and its two sister campgrounds, Fern Basin and Marion Mountain, are full. If so, drive to Idyllwild and go to the ranger station on the left as you enter town. They will direct you to dispersed camping areas. Some of these are "yellow post" areas, which means you can have a fire in the metal fire ring. Other areas require a fire permit, which will be issued at the station if fire conditions allow it.

Other alternatives include the two Mount San Jacinto State Park campgrounds. Idyllwild Campground is right smack in town by the Mount San Jacinto State Park Ranger Station. It is clean (flush toilets and showers), safe, and especially wonderful on Sunday morning, when you feel like walking 100 yards to Idyllwild for brunch and the Sunday paper. Many of Idyllwild's sites are for tents only, which makes the campground especially friendly. Stone Creek is out of town and a little more primitive.

Dark Canyon Campground

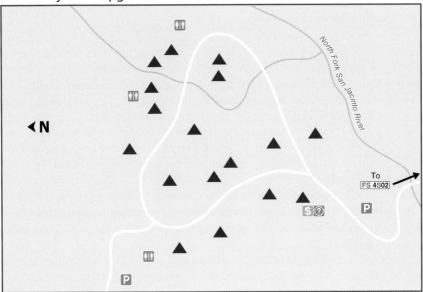

GETTING THERE

From Los Angeles, drive east on I-10 about 80 miles to Banning. Take CA 243 south 22 miles toward Idyllwild. Turn left on FS 4S02 and go another 3 miles to the campground.

GPS COORDINATES: N33° 48' 14" W116° 43' 56"

45

Hanna Flat Campground

Beauty ★★★★ / Privacy ★★★★★ / Spaciousness ★★★★★ / Quiet ★★★★★ / Security ★★★★★ / Cleanliness ★★★★★

With fishing, biking, and hiking options galore, Hanna Flat might be your heaven on earth, but don't venture here on big holidays.

"Abandon all hope, ye who enter here" is a good motto for campers coming to Big Bear Lake on holiday weekends, but during midweek or off-season, the north shore is downright civilized. It's a beautiful place, and the rangers and civilians are genuinely friendly.

Hanna Flat Campground features good tent camping. The sites are set in stands of Jeffrey pine and spaced nicely to allow vistas of pine-covered and rocky hills with the blue-sky, big-country look. Manzanita grows under the pines, and there's a mild riparian community by the cut along the campground. Best of all, the sites are engineered to give campers maximum privacy and space. Each site has an abundance of flat, spongy, and pine-needled ground.

Hanna Flat Campground is run by Alpine Camping Services, a private company, and they do a good job. When we visited Hanna Flat they were represented by a Grizzly Adams–type fellow in rawhide boots, and by his dad back at the camp host trailer. There are clean pit and flush toilets.

The few miles of dirt road coming in discourages most RVers, who prefer sites down by the lake in parks with hookups. In the nearby village of Fawnskin, you'll find a little grocery store and two homespun eateries. For serious shopping, go around the lake to

The view from site 63 indicates how popular this campground is.

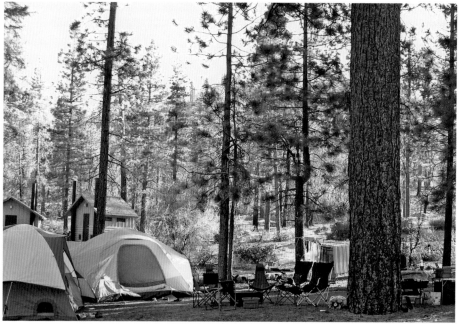

photographed by Patricia Frazier

KEY INFORMATION

LOCATION: Coxey Road, Fawnskin,
CA 92333

CONTACT: 909-382-2790,
www.fs.usda.gov/sbnf

OPERATED BY: California Land Management

OPEN: May 14–October 10

SITES: 86

EACH SITE: Picnic table, fire ring

ASSIGNMENT: Some sites offer reservations;
others are first come, first served

REGISTRATION: At entrance or reserve at
recreation.gov or 877-444-6777

FACILITIES: Water, flush toilets,
firewood for sale

PARKING: At site, additional vehicles
$5 per day

FEE: $27–$29 plus $9 nonrefundable
reservation fee

ELEVATION: 7,000'

RESTRICTIONS:

PETS: On leash only

FIRES: In fire ring

ALCOHOL: No restrictions

VEHICLES: RVs up to 40 feet;
fee for second vehicle

OTHER: 14-day stay limit

Big Bear City. There's a Thrifty as big as an aircraft carrier and more banks than you can shake a stick at.

Lake access from Hanna Flat Campground begins in Captain John's Fawn Harbor & Marina, which has a bait shop, a lake beach, picnic areas, and boat rentals. A sign announces roosting bald eagles from November to March. Fawnskin is charming. I loved all the rustic wood cottages.

More lake access lies below Serrano Campground, a few miles east of Fawnskin. There's a marina that rents boats and bicycles, an observatory, a paved hiking and biking path, and Meadow's Edge Picnic Area, with all the amenities and a nice lake beach. The observatory dome is out on the water at the end of a dock. Noted for its study of the sun, the observatory is open to the public Saturdays during July and August, 4–6 p.m.

Just past Serrano Campground is the Big Bear Ranger Station, where you can get maps of all the hiking trails. Big Bear offers good hiking and is a world-renowned mountain-biking center. Snow Summit, a snow-ski resort, utilizes its chairlifts in the summer to carry mountain bikers to the top of the mountain, at 8,200 feet, where there are 60 miles of accessible trails. The real fanatics go down Snow Summit's singletrack downhills at about 90 miles per hour.

Back at the Hanna Flat Campground, you'll find two fun hikes; one heads out from site 51 to Grout Bay Picnic Area, and the other goes from site 25 north and back along the road. The trail to Grout Bay is an 8-mile round-trip with lovely views of the lake from the plateau. Look for eagles on the tops of dead trees. From this trail, you can also access the trail to Gray's Peak. The trail is a bit rough as you near the summit.

The second hike takes you north to the beaver dams on Holcomb Creek. Here, beavers live in dens in caves along the water's edge. To more easily access the dams, drive your car out of the campground, turn left on the dirt road you came in on (FS 3N14), and go a mile or so to a parking lot on the right before Holcomb Creek. Find the Pacific Crest Trail just north across the creek and to the left of FS 3N14. Follow the trail west about a mile to see the beaver dams. Look for wildflowers along the way. I was able to identify wild rose, lupine, Indian paintbrush, and scarlet bugler.

Look at the mountains around Big Bear Lake and imagine—this was once the bottom of the ocean! Of course, that was about 600 million years ago. Then, 60 million years ago, the earth's plates ground together and pushed the ocean floor up to make the San Bernardinos.

The Big Bear Lake area can get crowded, so time your visits for maximum enjoyment. As you drive up the mountains to Big Bear, remember the area's first tourists, who rode for two days on burros up to the Bear Valley Hotel.

On the way home, drive the Rim of the World Highway (CA 18) to Redlands. Built in 1915, this road provided the first automobile access to Big Bear (no more burros!). The scenery is sensational.

Hanna Flat Campground

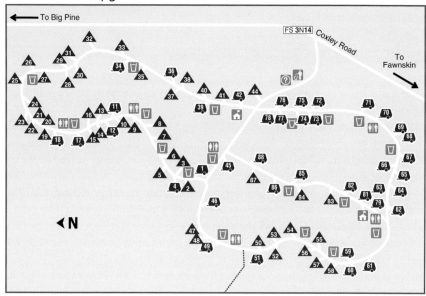

GETTING THERE

From Los Angeles, go east on I-10, almost to San Bernardino. Then take CA 30 north to CA 330. About 35 miles later, you will arrive at the Big Bear Lake dam. Go left on CA 38 for 4 miles to Fawnskin. Turn left on Rim of the World Drive. It becomes FS 3N14. Follow this dirt road a couple of miles to Hanna Flat Campground on the left.

GPS COORDINATES: N34° 17' 17" W116° 58' 33"

46

Heart Bar Campground

Beauty ★★★★ / Privacy ★★★★ / Spaciousness ★★★★ / Quiet ★★★★★ / Security ★★★★ / Cleanliness ★★★★★

This is real mountain camping right near Los Angeles.

Drive up to Big Bear on CA 330 and you feel like a rat in a maze. The road zips up through carnival-ride corners shouldered with impenetrable chaparral. Oncoming traffic appears out of nowhere. Suddenly, behind you, there's a string of impatient cars. You pull over, and they fly by in a flash of waxed paint and chrome.

You'll find a different scene on CA 38. Drive out of Big Bear into a sea of granite and lodgepole pine and feast your eyes on Old Greyback himself, San Gorgonio Mountain at 11,502 feet (named for an obscure Christian martyr). Come up from the bottom, from Redlands down in the desert, and suddenly you are in subalpine (boreal) forests of lodgepole pine twisted by the storms. The chaparral is high-altitude chaparral. There's manzanita, bush chinquapin, and snowbrush, plus all the alpine wildflowers. It's incredible!

Heart Bar Campground is right in the center of the San Gorgonio Wilderness. Why the name Heart Bar? It's a beautiful name. Here, in an area settled by pioneer Mormons, cattle herds were summered up in the meadows by the headwaters of the Santa Ana River. One of the local brands was the Heart Bar, a heart with a bar beneath it.

I love this campground. It's big and shaded but feels wide open. The meadow is green and bright in the sunlight. The pitches are clean and softened by pine needles. The sites are nicely spaced. And, the campground is not nearly as heavily used as nearby South Fork Campground, bunched along Lost Creek, or Barton Flats down below.

Just a short hike away, a remote meadow offers further escape.

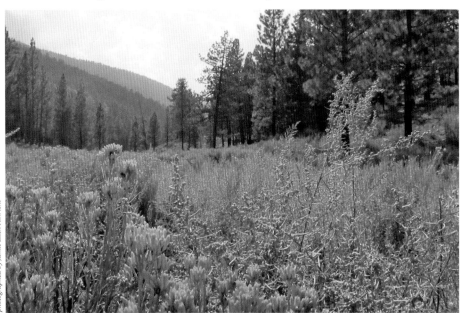

photographed by Jamie Ellen Hinrichs

KEY INFORMATION

LOCATION: CA 38 and FS 1N02,
Angelus Oaks, CA 92305

CONTACT: 909-382-2790,
www.fs.usda.gov/sbnf

OPERATED BY: California Land Management

OPEN: May 15–October 1

SITES: 95

EACH SITE: Picnic table, fire ring

ASSIGNMENT: Some sites offer reservations;
others are first come, first served

REGISTRATION: At entrance (or with host) or
reserve at recreation.gov or 877-444-6777

FACILITIES: Water, vault toilets

PARKING: At site, additional vehicles
$5 per night

FEE: $23–$25 plus $9 nonrefundable reservation fee; no fee for hiking, but auto touring
costs $5 per day or $30 annually

ELEVATION: 7,000'

RESTRICTIONS:

PETS: On leash only

FIRES: In fire pits

ALCOHOL: No restrictions

VEHICLES: RVs up to 50 feet

OTHER: Get a wilderness permit from Mill
Creek Ranger Station. Reserve for big
holidays.

There is great hiking from the campground, stream fishing down by the South Fork Campground, and lake fishing a short shot up at Big Bear Lake. At Big Bear, you can buy anything a body could need from big chain stores and little antique joints. Or, the other way, in Angelus Oaks, there's a general store as well as the Oaks Restaurant. You can also go farther and then left along Mill Creek to Forest Falls, where there is another general store.

For an easily accessed hike, head south a few hundred yards from Heart Bar Campground and connect with a trail that goes east to the headwaters of the Santa Ana River or west along its banks to South Fork Campground. Up here, the Santa Ana is a beautiful little stream flowing through meadows and forests of black oak, fir, and Jeffrey and ponderosa pine. Formed from natural springs and snowmelt, the Santa Ana River looks incredibly beautiful up here, yet hideously ugly down in Orange County in its concrete channel.

Or, hike up Wildhorse Creek. Walk out to the main road and go left. About 300 yards along you'll see a signed turnoff to the Wildhorse Trail on the right. Follow the dirt road up to a parking lot. The trail leaves from here. At first, it is an old road up through pines and juniper. Then it winds up a series of chaparral-covered ridges before going down into Wildhorse Creek Canyon. Walk about a mile and find Wildhorse Creek Trail Camp. Right now, you are about 3.5 miles out.

An ambitious hiker could continue and climb Sugar Loaf Mountain. Sugar Loaf has an elevation of about 9,952 feet and is a big lump on the divide between Big Bear country and the Santa Ana River Canyon. The best way is to hike up the saddle east of Sugar Loaf, then follow the trail along the ridgetop to the summit. I kept hearing about a famous, rare black butterfly and looked in vain for it when I was last there.

Another fun hike from Heart Bar Campground is to Aspen Grove. Go in the fall when the leaves are golden yellow. Head out of the campground to FS 1N02 (the road you drove in on). Turn right and walk about a mile to a fork in the road. Go right again and walk to a small parking lot near the signed trailhead for Aspen Grove Trail. Follow the old dirt road southeast to Fish Creek. Cross the creek and enjoy the aspens—or what's left of them.

Apparently, the California golden beaver enjoys them, too. A fellow hiker said that this particular beaver is not a San Bernardino native but was introduced by U.S. Forest Service wildlife experts who had not counted on the beaver's sudden passion for eating aspen.

Check out the dispersed camping in the area for future trips. Stop at the Mill Creek Ranger Station on CA 38 near the burg of Mentone. You'll need a wilderness permit for ambitious hiking anyway. Ask the ranger to show you where dispersed camping is allowed and where the yellow-post sites are. There is spectacular tent camping in the San Gorgonio area, and much of it is outside the organized campgrounds.

Heart Bar Campground

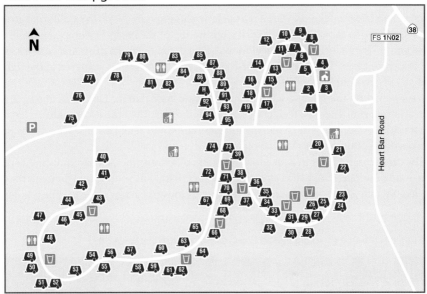

GETTING THERE

From Los Angeles, go east on I-10 about 62 miles to Redlands past San Bernardino. Then take CA 38 east 33 miles to FS 1N02 and turn right. The campground entrance is immediately on your right.

GPS COORDINATES: N34° 9' 41" W116° 47' 8"

47

Laguna Campground

Beauty ★★★★★ / Privacy ★★★★ / Spaciousness ★★★★ / Quiet ★★★★★ / Security ★★★★★ / Cleanliness ★★★★★

Laguna Campground is clean, well run, and near the proud community of Laguna.

Laguna Campground offers some of the best camping in Southern California and the cheekiest ground squirrels and jays in the West. Hardly had my wife and I arrived at an incredible campsite on the edge of a yellow-flowered meadow stretching away to islands of pine against a cerulean blue sky, when a larcenous Stellar's jay swooped down on the picnic table and tried to take off with a particularly shiny spoon. Next, the California ground squirrels moved in for a package of corn chips on top of the cooler. I stomped my feet and threw gravel. They scurried a few feet away, rolled defiantly in the dust, and rose to attack the corn chips again. Then, I heard a shrill shriek, and the varmints scattered at the sight of a red-tailed hawk circling above.

Maintained by the Laguna Mountain Volunteer Association, Laguna Campground is clean and well run. There's a feeling of serenity and order. The little community of Laguna, with its stores, churches, fire department, restaurants, and rental cabins, reflects the pride of its residents. This is a very special place.

The campground is set in a meadow in a stand of Jeffrey pines, almost indistinguishable from ponderosa pines, save the vanilla scent of their bark. Put your nose right up to the tree and take a whiff. Also, the bark on the Jeffrey tends toward narrow ridges, while ponderosa

Little Laguna Lake (in the background) becomes more of a marsh in summer.

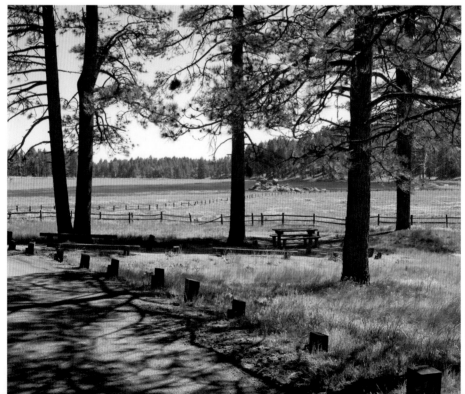

photographed by Bob Perry

KEY INFORMATION

LOCATION: Los Huecos Road,
Mt. Laguna, CA 91948

CONTACT: Ranger Office: 619-445-6235 or
619-473-8824 (Monday–Friday, 8 a.m.–
4:30 p.m.); visitor center: 619-473-8547
(Friday–Sunday, May–September); or
www.fs.usda.gov/cleveland

OPERATED BY: U.S. Forest Service

OPEN: Year-round

SITES: 104 total; 30 tent-only

EACH SITE: Picnic table, fire ring

ASSIGNMENT: Some sites offer reservations;
others are first come, first served

REGISTRATION: At entrance or reserve at
recreation.gov or 877-444-6777

FACILITIES: Water, vault toilets, showers

PARKING: Near site, additional vehicles
$8 per day

FEE: $22 plus $9 nonrefundable
reservation fee

ELEVATION: 5,800'

RESTRICTIONS:

PETS: On leash only and must stay in tent
or vehicle at night

FIRES: In fire pit

ALCOHOL: No restrictions

VEHICLES: RVs up to 25 feet, trailers

bark grows in large, flat plates. Roll the cones from a Jeffrey between your hands, and the spines won't prick—they are turned under. Ponderosa spines stick out.

American Indians used the roots of Jeffrey pines to make baskets. They waited until the trees flowered and the roots were sufficiently tough. Then, they dug up the roots, cleaned, and slow-cooked them. Afterward, the roots were split and scraped until soft and pliable enough to weave.

I met a German naturalist camping a few sites over who gave me the rundown on the squirrels. They are supposed to eat seeds, herbaceous vegetation, and acorns, but prefer to hang around campgrounds and eat corn chips. They hibernate in the winter; when spring comes, they have some catch-up eating to do. According to the naturalist, the shrill squeak I heard when the hawk cruised overhead was from the oldest squirrel in the colony. Apparently, the squirrel who sounds the alarm has the greatest chance of being picked off by the hawk. So, the oldest squirrel protects his own offspring, and the band, by sounding the alarm and offering himself as the victim if need be. Pretty brave stuff for the little guy.

In the meadow by the campground is Little Laguna Lake. Little more than a wallow, it is still home to many waterfowl and loudly croaking frogs. A kopje (a stand of rocks in a meadow) nearby is a convenient place to sit and watch the wildlife through binoculars. When I visited in June, the meadow was carpeted with tiny sunflowers, tidy tips, Achilles's fern, and the edible miner's lettuce.

We picked up a trail to Big Laguna Lake from the south of the campground. The trail meanders for about a mile across meadows and along the edge of the pined hummocks that beg for picnickers. Big Laguna Lake, which is only a lake indeed in the spring and summer of wet years, was big and beautiful on our visit. From the lake, the mostly flat trail turns north and connects with Noble Canyon Trail and Pine Creek Road.

If you want a desert view, trade the pines of Laguna for the oaks of Burnt Rancheria Campground a few miles south, also run by the Laguna Mountain Volunteer Society.

Laguna Campground is open all year (Burnt Rancheria is open May to October), but I think spring is the best time to visit. In winter, there's snow and snow sports, but half of San

Diego flocks here on wintry weekends. Summers get a bit hot and dusty. Both campgrounds are popular, so plan on getting here Friday by noon if you don't have a reservation.

While visiting, run down to Tecate, Mexico (30 minutes to the south). Or, take I-8 to Anza-Borrego Desert State Park or the Sunrise Highway north to Julian to fish in Lake Cuyamaca. There is a lot to do around here. Go horseback riding or mountain biking. Stargaze from the night-sky observatories at the south end of the recreation area. This is a wonderful part of Southern California.

Laguna Campground

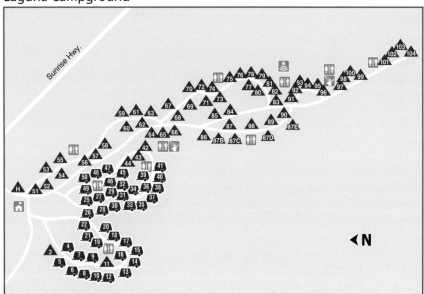

GETTING THERE

From San Diego, drive 50 miles east on I-8 to the Laguna Junction exit. Drive 11 miles farther north on Sunrise Highway to Mount Laguna, then 2.5 miles north to the signed entrance on the left marked Laguna/El Prado. Laguna is the campground you want.

GPS COORDINATES: N32 ° 53' 17" W116° 26' 57"

48

Marion Mountain Campground

Beauty ★★★ / Privacy ★★★★★ / Spaciousness ★★★★★ / Quiet ★★★★★ / Security ★★★★★ / Cleanliness ★★★★★

Marion Mountain, nestled in the clouds, is a great break from nearby Los Angeles.

From Los Angeles, the ride to Marion Mountain Campground on I-10 through the Inland Empire (also known as the Land of Swirling Gases) is an unsightly urban metropolis that never seems to end. Persevere, though, and head up CA 243 from Banning, and, in a few short minutes, you'll be in a different world. You'll come up out of the chaparral into the pines and peaks. What a contrast!

Marion Mountain Campground is as sunny and airy as nearby Dark Canyon Campground is dark and safe, down under sheltering trees. Between the two, you'll see the entire spectrum of good San Jacinto tent camping.

The access road to Marion Mountain Campground from CA 243 is narrow and winding. This cuts down on the trailers and RVs. The site parking spaces are short—about 15 feet tops. The picnic tables and fire pits are down in the trees away from the parking area. All this discourages RVers and gives an edge to tent campers.

The water from a spring above the campground is good. Let the tap run for a moment to clear any sediment if the campground has been lightly used. All the facilities are well maintained. The pit-toilet bathrooms are surprisingly clean, with tile floors and walls. I wanted to stay for a week. When you first arrive at Marion Mountain Campground, it's difficult to

Take the Marion Mountain Trail to one of the signature features of San Bernardino National Forest.

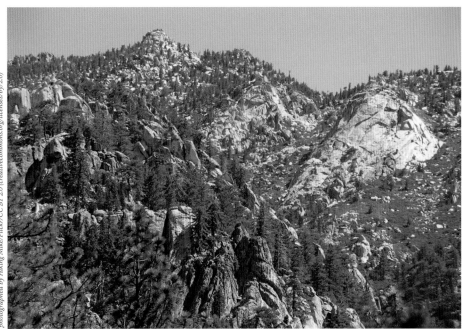

KEY INFORMATION

LOCATION: Marion Mountain Campground Road, Idyllwild-Pine Cove, CA 92549

CONTACT: 909-382-2921, www.fs.usda.gov/sbnf

OPERATED BY: U.S. Forest Service

OPEN: May–mid-October

SITES: 24

EACH SITE: Picnic table, fire ring

ASSIGNMENT: Some sites offer reservations; others are first come, first served

REGISTRATION: At entrance or reserve at recreation.gov or 877-444-6777

FACILITIES: Water, pit toilets

PARKING: Near site, additional vehicles $5 per day

FEE: $10 plus $9 nonrefundable reservation fee

ELEVATION: 6,400'

RESTRICTIONS:

PETS: On leash only

FIRES: In fire pit

ALCOHOL: No restrictions

VEHICLES: RVs up to 15 feet

OTHER: No dogs allowed within Mount San Jacinto State Park wilderness; permits are required to enter wilderness.

locate the sites. This is because most of them are isolated from each other among the pines. The pitches, on pine needles, are nice and spongy. Through the pine boughs, you'll see the steep slopes of the mountains across the canyon, all covered with pines, oaks, and rocky tors.

To hike from the campground, go to site 12. Across from that site's picnic table, there is a dirt road that heads up the slope. Follow it for 20 yards and notice the trail arrows pointing right and left. The right arrows lead you down the hill to the trailhead. The left ones indicate the Marion Mountain Trail, which goes up into the state park and joins the Pacific Crest Trail near Deer Spring. It climbs the heavily forested northwest flank of Marion Mountain and is the shortest way to climb San Jacinto Peak.

Take plenty of water and be aware of thunderstorms. When there is lightning, avoid open areas like meadows, ridges, and mountaintops. Stay away from isolated trees and take cover under dense, small trees in lower areas, in a boulder field, or in a cave. Failing all this, lie flat on the ground. And, in all cases, remove metal-frame backpacks and metal tent poles. Really, lightning is no joke. I suffered a near miss in the Mojave Desert a few summers ago. It burned my calves and scared me half to death.

In early September, when I last visited Marion Mountain, thunderstorm clouds appeared over the mountains. The dry air carried a hint of rain. As we were hiking up the slopes around the campground, there was a roll of thunder, and a splatter of rain hit the dusty rocks. What drama! The campground host told me they'd had a hard storm hit in the middle of August. It rained like hell for a couple of hours, and then the sun came out. This is typical of the Southern Sierras in late August and September, and something to watch for.

A good place for a sundowner is up the dirt road across from site 12. Go past the arrows for the Marion Mountain Trail. About 20 yards up, climb the ridge to the right, and there are some nice big boulders to sit on and watch the sun set. Back on the dirt road, walk to the end of it. There's a short trail that switchbacks up the slope to some cabins, where there is an incredible view of the southwest side of the range.

Head south to Pine Cove to find gas and ice. For a town with everything, go a few miles farther to Idyllwild, a lovely little mountain town. Idyllwild even has a shopping center with a supermarket and a hardware store. They have butchers, restaurants, artists, writers, and the San Jacinto Ranger Station—to the left as you enter town. If Marion Mountain and the other campgrounds nearby are full, or if you want to disperse-camp or yellow-post-camp, that's where you need to go. The rangers will fix you up with a fire permit and show you where to go.

Marion Mountain Campground

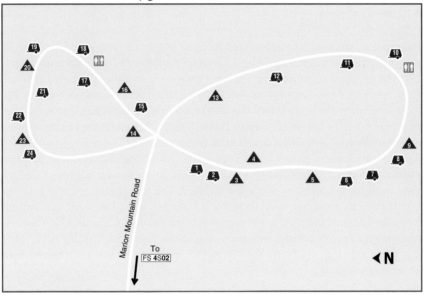

GETTING THERE

From Los Angeles, take I-10 east 84 miles to Banning. Go south on CA 243 for 22 miles. Turn left at FS 4S02 and drive 1.7 miles to the campground.

GPS COORDINATES: N33° 47' 31" W116° 43' 54"

49

Palomar Mountain State Park:
DOANE VALLEY CAMPGROUND

Beauty ★★★ / Privacy ★★★★ / Spaciousness ★★★ / Quiet ★★★ / Security ★★★★★ / Cleanliness ★★★★

See the stars at Palomar Observatory, eat at Mother's Kitchen Restaurant, and bring home 10 pounds of gems.

Palomar means "place of the pigeons," and Palomar Mountain State Park feels so Mediterranean, you'll think you're in Italy. There's a sense of tradition and civilization on the mountain. Maybe that feeling comes from the fact that American Indians gathered acorns here long ago, or drifts down from the incredible handcrafted observatory on the summit. Or maybe it stems from the sense of awe that observatory visitors get when they realize we live in but a tiny part of the universe. Anyway, Doane Valley Campground at Palomar Mountain State Park offers good tent camping and great family camping.

Built by the Civilian Conservation Corps in the 1930s (when folks camped in tents and cars were tiny Fords), the campsites are styled in stone and set under huge trees. The toilets are clean, and the hot showers cost a few quarters. The park headquarters is back up the road on the way in, and when I was there it was staffed by a helpful ranger who looked like a young Elke Sommer. Included in the park area is the Palomar Christian Conference Center and youth camps, all infested with boisterous junior high schoolers. If you tire of camp grub, at the intersection of County Road S6 and S7, you'll find Mother's Kitchen Restaurant, which serves good food.

In the early 1880s George Edwin Doane settled here in a shake-roof log cabin between Upper and Lower Doane Valley. Now, campers enjoy the same scenery.

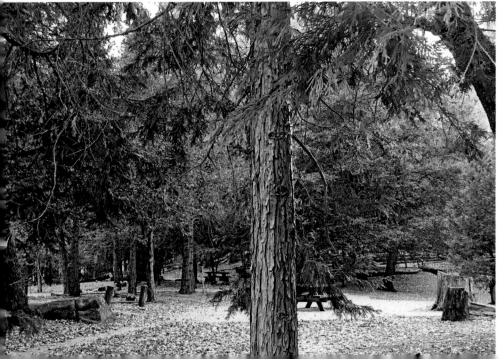

photographed by VALEEHILL

KEY INFORMATION

LOCATION: 19952 State Park Road, Palomar Mountain, CA 92060

CONTACT: 760-742-3462, parks.ca.gov; for information on neighboring Cleveland National Forest call 858-673-6180 or visit www.fs.usda.gov/cleveland

OPERATED BY: California State Parks

OPEN: Year-round

SITES: 31

EACH SITE: Picnic table, fire ring

ASSIGNMENT: First come, first served or by reservation

REGISTRATION: At entrance or reserve at reservecalifornia.com or 800-444-7275

FACILITIES: Water, flush toilets, coin-operated hot showers, firewood for sale, wheelchair-accessible sites

PARKING: Near site

FEE: $30 plus $8 nonrefundable reservation fee

ELEVATION: 4,700'

RESTRICTIONS:

PETS: On leash only (not allowed on trails)

FIRES: In fire pit; may be prohibited during high fire danger

ALCOHOL: No restrictions

VEHICLES: RVs up to 27 feet

OTHER: Stay limit of 7 consecutive days; 30 days annually; no off-road travel

---

Near the campground is Doane's Pond, a cute pond with picnic tables set around it under ramadas, because it gets hot here in the summer. On the road in, you'll see a sign threatening a $500 fine for miscreants throwing snowballs at cars or people, so you know snow drifts up a bit here in the winter. I think the best time to visit is in the spring or fall. But, the Palomar Observatory qualifies the mountain as a wonderful place to visit year-round. I think it's easier to view ourselves as creatures of the larger universe when camping than when being on our computers at home. Buy the star map in the observatory gift shop and go out in the meadow by Doane's Pond at night. Imagine how the ancients must have felt in a world lit only by starlight and fire.

I followed a group of junior high schoolers and heard their teacher try to pique the loutish pupils' interest in the observatory. It really is amazing. The dome weighs 1,000 tons and is so well engineered that it can be moved by hand. The telescope, which weighs 750 tons, can also be moved by the touch of a finger. The glass disk at the heart of the telescope was ground and polished to the two-millionth part of an inch. Incredible!

It wasn't hard to spot the band-tailed pigeon that gives Palomar Mountain its name. The band-tail is not your ordinary "rat with wings" pigeon cadging food at the local patio restaurant, but a lovely bird with a yellow bill, green nape, and white neckband. Its call is a low-pitched, owl-like "coo-coo."

Like the band-tail, the acorn woodpecker eats acorns. It goes around storing them by the thousands in specially drilled holes—each containing a single acorn—in dead trees, telephone poles, fence posts, and even the sides of buildings. Its diligence is equaled only by the gray squirrel, which hides acorns in underground caches and later smells them out. Acorns are a big industry on the mountain.

The Luiseno tribe, who also collected acorns on Palomar, ate manzanita berries, choke cherries, and toyon berries. For salad and veggies, they ate lily bulbs, tree mushrooms, yucca blossoms, sage shoots, wild mustard, clover, and celery. In season, they relished watercress, lamb's quarter, and Indian lettuce. Palomar is a bountiful mountain.

If you don't find a site at Doane Valley Campground (reserve ahead for weekends!), there are two U.S. Forest Service camps up the road to the observatory. At wide-open Observatory Campground there are huge oaks and views of the ridges. Just 0.25 mile up is Fry Creek Campground, a nice campground in the woods that favors tent campers because the road in is too narrow for RVs or trailers.

A good side trip from Palomar is to Gems of Pala, just down the road toward I-15. It's open Thursday through Sunday, 10 a.m. to 4 p.m. For a fee, you get to dig in one of the world's foremost tourmaline locations. Bring a garden shovel, a spray bottle, and a one-eighth-inch mesh screen about one foot by two feet. You get to take home up to 10 pounds of pink, blue, green, black, and watermelon tourmaline. Call Gems of Pala at 760-742-1356 for information.

Doane Valley Campground

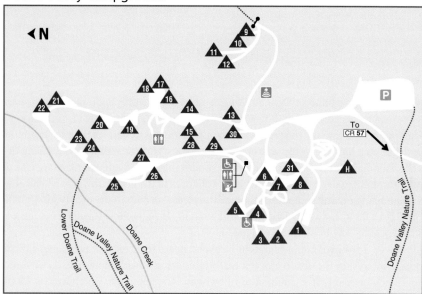

GETTING THERE

From Los Angeles take I-10 east about 40 miles to I-15. Take I-15 south about 62 miles to the intersection with CA 76. Drive east 21 miles to County Road S6. Go north (left) 6.8 miles, then turn left on CR S7 and 3 miles to the campground.

GPS COORDINATES: N 33° 20' 38" W116° 54' 04"

50

William Heise County Park Campground

Beauty ★★★★ / Privacy ★★ / Spaciousness ★★★ / Quiet ★★★ / Security ★★★ / Cleanliness ★★★

Visit California high country and feel like you're in Vermont at the same time.

Among the many reasons to camp in William Heise County Park are the incredible drives in from Los Angeles via Warner Springs or from San Diego via Ramona or Cuyamaca Rancho State Park. All show Southern California at its most charming and very best—the rolling, forested hills; the green meadows; and the tiny western towns. This was the real gold the forty-niners found when they arrived in California—this beautiful land. On all three drives, near Julian, you climb 2 miles south on Pine Hills Road, then turn left on Frisius Drive. Those final 2 miles carry you through farmland that echoes bucolic Vermont or New Hampshire. The resemblance is eerie.

Made up of 929 acres of oak, pine, and cedar, William Heise County Park is upper chaparral; this area is also known as cold chaparral because most of the precipitation comes from snow and fog drip. As you hike around and in the park, watch the slope orientation to see the effect.

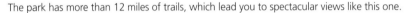

The park has more than 12 miles of trails, which lead you to spectacular views like this one.

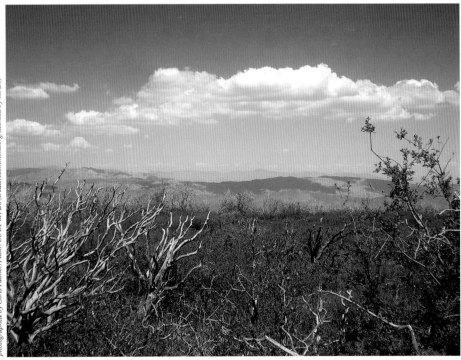

photographed by Chris Palmer/Flickr/CC BY-SA 2.0 (creativecommons.org/licenses/by-sa/2.0)

KEY INFORMATION

LOCATION: 4945 Heise Park Road, Julian, CA 92036

OPERATED BY: San Diego County Department of Parks and Recreation

CONTACT: 760-765-0650, sdparks.org

OPEN: Year-round

SITES: 103

EACH SITE: Picnic table, fire ring, tent pad, water nearby

ASSIGNMENT: First come, first served; reservations recommended

REGISTRATION: By entrance; for reservations call 858-565-3600 or visit reservations.sdparks.org

FACILITIES: Water, flush toilets, showers, playground

PARKING: At individual sites

FEE: $29, $5 nonrefundable reservation fee

ELEVATION: 4,200'

RESTRICTIONS:

PETS: On 6-foot leash; must be attended at all times; $1 fee; not allowed on hiking trails

FIRES: In fire ring

VEHICLES: RVs, small trailers

ALCOHOL: Beer and wine; nothing over 40-proof

OTHER: Check-in time is noon, checkout is 2 p.m.; $3 per vehicle for day-use parking

On south-facing slopes you'll see evergreen shrubs with thick oval leaves, such as the manzanita. Note how the manzanita leaves are mealy and waxy and are often oriented vertically to reduce the amount of light that directly strikes the leaf surface. Manzanita endure droughts, resist fire, and withstand cold. On north-facing slopes look for California live oak; Jeffrey, Coulter, sugar, and ponderosa pines; white fir; and incense cedar.

Like Cuyamaca Rancho State Park, William Heise is a birder's paradise. Look for various hawks, eagles, owls, woodpeckers, vireos, warblers, sparrows, and the like. Also look for the full complement of Southern California reptiles and various rodents eating the plethora of acorns. Acorns were a Cahuilla Indian staple, made into meal and then bread.

Once, camping at William Heise, we experimented with acorn bread. First, we ground the acorns into a coarse meal, then, following a local Cahuilla recipe, we filled a colander with fine sand, patted the coarsely ground acorn meal down into a bowl-like depression in the sand, and poured water slowly over the meal to leach out the bitterness. Then we pounded the meal down in a mortar until it resembled a fine powder. Finally, the meal was sifted, mixed with water, and baked on a hot rock: not bad, but a little bitter.

Heise is a friendly place to camp. Almost half of the sites are for tents only. The park is roomy, and the restrooms are very clean. Once, we rented one of the cabins at Heise. It had six wooden bunks and a maximum capacity of six ($62 per night plus $5 reservation fee). Bring your own bedding and a padlock for the door. Cooking is done outside on a grill.

Heise is a fine base camp from which to explore Julian, Wynola, and Santa Ysabel. Stop for a drink or breakfast at the much-fabled Pine Hills Lodge on La Posada Way in Julian. Visit the Santa Ysabel Mission 2 miles north of Santa Ysabel on CA 79. See the museum in Julian. Take the Eagle Mine tour. Ask the ranger or campground host at Heise about trips to Boulder Creek and Boulder Creek Falls. Don't miss a killer hike (11 miles round-trip) down Kelly Ditch Trail to Cuyamaca Rancho State Park.

William Heise County Park Campground

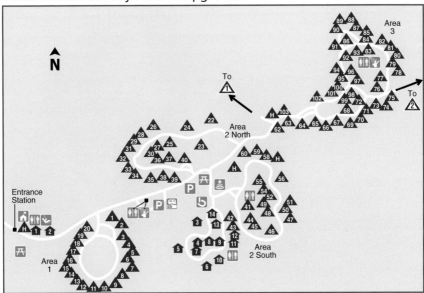

GETTING THERE

From Los Angeles, take I-10 east about 40 miles to I-15. Go south on I-15 about 50 miles to Temecula. Take CA 79 southeast 53 miles to Santa Ysabel. Turn left to continue on CA 79 toward Julian for 5.8 miles to Pine Hills Road. Turn right and drive 2 miles to Frisius Drive. Turn left and drive 2 miles to the park. (Frisius Drive turns into Heise Park Road near the park.)

GPS COORDINATES: N33° 02' 25" W116° 35' 19"

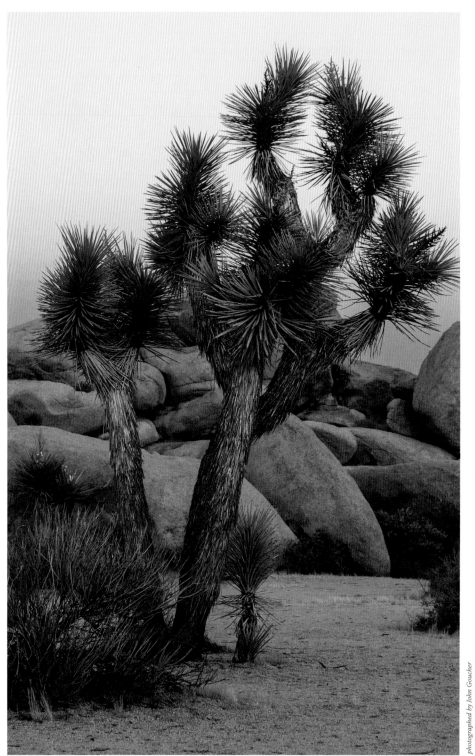

At White Tank Campground, located within Joshua Tree National Park, Joshua trees are a common sight (see page 56).

APPENDIX A

CAMPING EQUIPMENT CHECKLIST

Except for the large and bulky items on this list, I keep a plastic storage container full of the essentials of car camping so that they're ready to go when I am. I make a last-minute check of the inventory and resupply anything that's low or missing, and away I go.

COOKING UTENSILS

Bottle opener
Bottles of salt, pepper, spices, sugar, cooking oil, and maple syrup in waterproof, spill-proof containers
Can opener
Corkscrew
Cups, plastic or tin
Dish soap (biodegradable), sponge, towel
Flatware
Food of your choice
Frying pan
Fuel for stove
Matches in waterproof container
Plates
Pocketknife
Pot with lid
Spatula
Stove
Tin foil
Wooden spoon

FIRST AID KIT

Adhesive bandages
Antibiotic cream
Aspirin or ibuprofen
Diphenhydramine (Benadryl)
Gauze pads
Insect repellent
Moleskin
Snakebite kit (if you're heading for desert conditions)
Sunscreen/lip balm
Tape, waterproof adhesive
Tweezers

SLEEPING GEAR

Pillow
Sleeping bag
Sleeping pad (inflatable or insulated)
Tent with ground tarp and rainfly

MISCELLANEOUS

Bath soap (biodegradable), washcloth, towel
Camp chair
Candles
Cellular phone
Cooler
Deck of cards
Fire starter
Flashlight or headlamp with fresh batteries
Foul-weather clothing (useful year-round in the Northwest)
Lantern
Paper towels
Plastic zip-top bags
Sunglasses
Toilet paper
Water bottle
Wool blanket

OPTIONAL

Barbecue grill
Binoculars
Field guides on bird, plant, and wildlife identification
Fishing rod and tackle
GPS
Hatchet
Maps (road, topographic, trails, etc.)

APPENDIX B

SUGGESTED READING AND REFERENCE

Braden, Otie. *Gem Trails of Southern California.* Upland, CA: Gem Guides Book Co., 2017.

Chase, J. Smeaton. *California Desert Trails.* N.p., 2017.

Harris, David. *Afoot & Afield Inland Empire.* Birmingham, AL: Wilderness Press, 2018.

Irwin, Sue. *California's Eastern Sierra.* Los Olivos, CA: Cachuma Press, 1992.

Lindsay, Lowell and Diana. *Anza-Borrego Desert Region.* Birmingham, AL: Wilderness Press, 2018.

Robinson, John W. and David Harris. *San Bernardino Mountain Trails.* Birmingham, AL: Wilderness Press, 2016.

Schoenherr, Allan A. *A Natural History of California.* Berkeley, CA: University of California Press, 1995.

Stienstra, Tom. *California Camping.* Berkeley, CA: Moon Outdoors, 2017.

APPENDIX C

SOURCES OF INFORMATION

BLM, CALIFORNIA STATE HEADQUARTERS
Bureau of Land Management
State Government Office
Susanville, CA
530-257-0456
ca.blm.gov

CALIFORNIA STATE PARKS
PO Box 942896
Sacramento, CA 94296
916-653-6995
parks.ca.gov

DEATH VALLEY NATIONAL PARK
PO Box 579
Death Valley, CA 92328
760-786-3200
nps.gov/deva

INYO NATIONAL FOREST
351 Pacu Lane, Suite 200
Bishop, CA 93514
760-873-2400
www.fs.usda.gov/inyo

JOSHUA TREE NATIONAL PARK
74485 National Park Drive
Twentynine Palms, CA 92277-3597
760-367-5500
nps.gov/jotr

LOS PADRES NATIONAL FOREST
6750 Navigator Way, Suite150
Goleta, CA 93117
805-968-6640
www.fs.usda.gov/lpnf

MOJAVE NATIONAL PRESERVE
2701 Barstow Road
Barstow, CA 92311
760-252-6100
nps.gov/moja

NATIONAL PARK SERVICE, PACIFIC WEST REGIONAL OFFICE
333 Bush Street, Suite 500
San Francisco, CA 94104-2828
415-623-2100
nps.gov

PINNACLES CAMPGROUND STORE
2400 Highway 146
Paicines, CA 95043
831-389-4462

PINNACLES NATIONAL PARK
5000 Highway 146
Paicines, CA 95043
831-389-4485
nps.gov/pinn

SAN BERNARDINO NATIONAL FOREST
602 South Tippecanoe Avenue
San Bernardino, CA 92408
909-382-2600
www.fs.usda.gov/sbnf

SEQUOIA & KINGS CANYON NATIONAL PARK
47050 Generals Highway
Three Rivers, CA 93271-9651
559-565-3341
nps.gov/seki

SEQUOIA NATIONAL FOREST
1839 South Newcomb Street
Porterville, CA 93257
559-784-1500
www.fs.usda.gov/sequoia

SIERRA NATIONAL FOREST
1600 Tollhouse Road
Clovis, CA 93611-0532
559-297-0706
www.fs.usda.gov/sierra

**U.S. FOREST SERVICE,
PACIFIC SOUTHWEST REGION**
1323 Club Drive
Vallejo, CA 94592
707-562-8737
www.fs.usda.gov/r5

YOSEMITE NATIONAL PARK
PO Box 577
Yosemite National Park, CA 95389
209-372-0200
nps.gov/yose

Trumbull Lake reflects its surrounding landscape (see page 130).

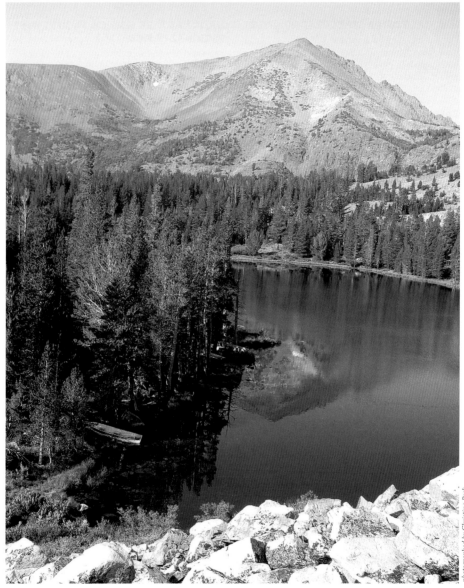

photographed by Christina Peck

INDEX

ABOUT THE AUTHOR

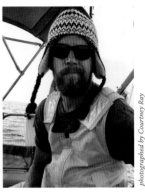

photographed by Courtney Ray

Charles Patterson, a Southern California native, daydreams about his next outdoor adventure every time he finds himself indoors, bound by some professional or otherwise mundane obligation. Naturally, he relishes the opportunity to explore further, pushing himself to greater lengths than most would tolerate. Writing _Mountain Bike! Los Angeles County: A Wide-Grin Ride Guide_ forced Charles to spend many hours in the sticks, often alone, occasionally pondering the size of local mountain lion populations. It was a true adventure, and getting to write about it afterward and share his love for the outdoors was a blessing. Revising _Best Tent Camping: Southern California_ is a natural progression because Charles's banged-up body certainly can't tolerate two-wheeled pursuits forever, and tent camping is an activity he'll still be able to enjoy after his first walker, cane, or wheelchair purchase.

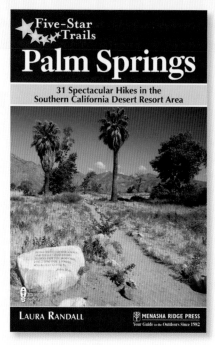

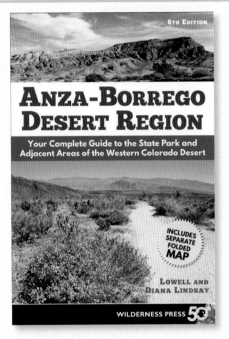

Check out this other great title from
— Menasha Ridge Press! —

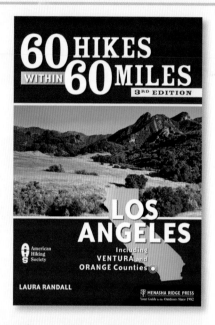

60 Hikes Within 60 Miles:
Los Angeles

by Laura Randall
ISBN: 978-1-63404-036-5
$18.95, 3rd Edition

6x9, paperback
maps, photographs, index

With time, health, and pin money at a premium, *60 Hikes Within 60 Miles: Los Angeles* helps Angelenos get back to nature without going out of town. From Palos Verdes on the coast to Santa Clarita to the north and the expansive San Gabriel Mountains, this guide details 60 hikes and walks within roughly an hour's drive of Los Angeles, encouraging even the most time-starved trekkers to get on the trails and get healthy.

Having lived in just about every area of Los Angeles, author Laura Randall provides key in-the-know information about traffic patterns, the best times to hike, how to avoid expensive parking fees, and the best burrito joints near the trailhead.

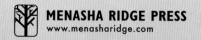

MENASHA RIDGE PRESS
www.menasharidge.com

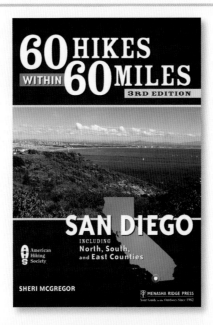
 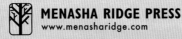

Check out this other great title from
Wilderness Press!

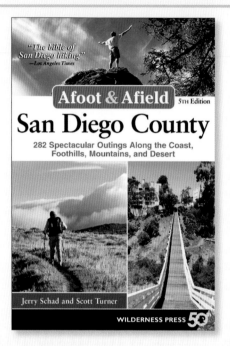

Afoot & Afield: San Diego County

by Jerry Schad & Scott Turner
ISBN: 978-0-89997-801-7
$24.95, 5th Edition

6x9, paperback
maps, photographs, index

Since 1986, Jerry Schad's *Afoot and Afield: San Diego County* has been the premier trail guide for hikers, backpackers, and mountain bikers. It describes routes ranging from brief, family-friendly hikes to multiple-day overnight trips in remote regions of the backcountry, providing equal weight to the scenic and recreational value of each trip. Each route features at least one or more significant botanical, cultural, or geological highlight with detailed information about what makes each one special. The book's lengthy history as the preferred hiking guide for the region creates trust and recognition in its readers, while the variety within the book caters to a wide population of recreational enthusiasts.

Current coauthor Scott Turner has fully updated the book by re-hiking each of the routes contained within the book and adding new routes to ensure that information for each trip is fully current.

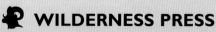 WILDERNESS PRESS

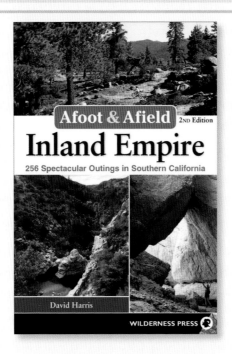
 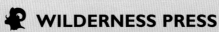

DEAR CUSTOMERS AND FRIENDS,

SUPPORTING YOUR INTEREST IN OUTDOOR ADVENTURE, travel, and an active lifestyle is central to our operations, from the authors we choose to the locations we detail to the way we design our books. Menasha Ridge Press was incorporated in 1982 by a group of veteran outdoorsmen and professional outfitters. For many years now, we've specialized in creating books that benefit the outdoors enthusiast.

Almost immediately, Menasha Ridge Press earned a reputation for revolutionizing outdoors- and travel-guidebook publishing. For such activities as canoeing, kayaking, hiking, backpacking, and mountain biking, we established new standards of quality that transformed the whole genre, resulting in outdoor-recreation guides of great sophistication and solid content. Menasha Ridge Press continues to be outdoor publishing's greatest innovator.

The folks at Menasha Ridge Press are as at home on a whitewater river or mountain trail as they are editing a manuscript. The books we build for you are the best they can be, because we're responding to your needs. Plus, we use and depend on them ourselves.

We look forward to seeing you on the river or the trail. If you'd like to contact us directly, visit us at menasharidge.com. We thank you for your interest in our books and the natural world around us all.

SAFE TRAVELS,

Bob Sehlinger

BOB SEHLINGER
PUBLISHER